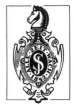

Offshore Medicine

Medical Care of Employees in the
Offshore Oil Industry

Second Edition

Edited by
R.A.F. Cox

Foreword by Ian McCallum

With 36 Figures

Springer-Verlag
London Berlin Heidelberg New York
Paris Tokyo

R.A.F. Cox, MA, MB, BChir, FFOM
Chief Medical Officer,
Central Electricity Generating Board.
Courtenay House,
18 Warwick Lane,
London EC4P 4EB

formerly Medical Director,
Phillips Petroleum Company Europe-Africa,
The Adelphi,
John Adam Street,
London WC2N 6BW

Library of Congress Cataloging-in-Publication Data. Offshore medicine.
Includes bibliographies and index.
1. Offshore oil industry – Hygienic aspects. 2. Petroleum workers – Diseases and
hygiene. 3. Offshore oil industry – Hygienic aspects – Great Britain. I. Cox, R.A.F.
(Robin Anthony Frederick), 1935-   . II. Anderson, I.K. [DNLM: 1. Occupational
Medicine. 2. Petroleum. WA 400 032] RC965.P48037 1986 362.1′088622 86-20345
ISBN-13: 978-1-4471-1397-3   e-ISBN-13: 978-1-4471-1395-9
DOI: 10.1007/ 978-1-4471-1395-9

Filmset by Computerised Typesetting Services Limited, 311 Ballards Lane, Finchley,
London NI2 8LY

2128/3916-543210

To Thomas and Clare, for whom this
book is especially significant

Foreword

To be asked to prepare a second edition of a book is heartening for any author or editor. Apart from the opportunity to make the corrections and amendments which are inevitable in a practical manual there is also the possibility to make additions which enhance its usefulness. Above all a further edition usually means that the book has been found to be acceptable to a large number of readers and has fulfilled a need. This is indeed the case with *Offshore Medicine,* which in its description of the medical aspects of offshore work has provided a unique guide to the occupational health of a new industry. The rapid development of offshore exploration for gas and oil which began in the 1960s created a whole new range of related industries. Most attention was focused on the problems of deep diving in the North Sea because of the great expansion of the diving industry, its technological advances and the high mortality of divers in the early years. Diving, however, is only a fraction of the total endeavour concerned with the offshore industry. The much larger population of workers offshore who man the rigs and barges, the toolpushers, helicopter pilots, crane drivers, scaffolders and roustabouts, geologists and so on, so sympathetically described by A. Alvarez in his recent book *Offshore, A North Sea Journey,* and the harsh and difficult conditions in which they often have to work are sometimes forgotten.

Offshore Medicine provides a valuable source of information for those concerned with the health and safety of everyone offshore. The contents of the book confirm the point made by Dr. Robin Cox that it describes a subspecialty of occupational medicine which is not covered by textbooks on that subject. Offshore work is referred to here as being characterised by 'frenetic activity and enormous costs'. Doctor, nurse and medic as part of that activity can contribute to it positively by good and soundly based advice related to offshore conditions. In this the industry is well served for not only is a fit man a good thing in itself, but in such difficult conditions the health and safety of others may depend on his fitness and effectiveness.

The range of problems covered here is wide, but particularly important is the description of the role of the general practitioner in offshore work and the importance of the flexibility which he can bring to it. This may on occasion lead to greater involvement in occupational medicine, as it has done in Dr. Cox's case, but the committed general practitioner who becomes involved in offshore work for part of his time will find a very valuable source of essential information here. The second edition maintains the qualities of the first and extends them.

R. IAN McCALLUM
MD, DSc, FRCP Lond, FRCP Ed, FFOM
Emeritus Professor of Occupational Health and Hygiene,
University of Newcastle upon Tyne,
Past Dean of the Faculty of Occupational Medicine,
Consultant, Institute of Occupational Medicine, Edinburgh

Preface to the First Edition

Offshore Medicine is hardly a speciality in its own right, but it is a part of occupational medicine which is so circumscribed that it may certainly be regarded as a sub-speciality. It covers all health matters which arise in connection with the exploration for and production of hydrocarbons from beneath the sea.

In whatever endeavours men may engage, whether voyages of exploration, cultivation of the land or manufacturing industry, there will be a mutual interaction between the enterprise and the health of the people engaged in it. The field of offshore engineering has been a frontier area since it began, just after the Second World War. The men in this rapidly growing technological area have been at the centre of a series of operations where human endeavour and engineering technology have been stretched to the limit by the hostile environment. In these circumstances, it is small wonder that health care in its broadest sense has required very special consideration.

Because of the ever-increasing need to search for further reserves of oil and gas, it is likely that deep water exploration will be extended to many areas of the world, where the local medical community may have no idea of the problems it is likely to have to face to satisfy this demanding industry. At the same time, the industry has an obligation to take care of its people as carefully and effectively as it can within the constraints of the operating conditions. It is to help the doctors, engineers, administrators and others who may be called upon to discharge this obligation that this book has been written.

When exploration of the southern North Sea commenced in the mid 1960s, no-one had seriously faced the health problems which this highly specialised industry posed. To some extent, this was because what little offshore exploration and development had been accomplished was in shallow water, relatively good weather conditions and often close to land. Furthermore, it had been conducted in an unobtrusive way, adjacent to areas where oil production on land was commonplace and familiar and where the peculiar demands of the industry were an everyday fact of life. The drilling in the North Sea was different. It was a new and unique experience for Great Britain and every aspect of the task was therefore newsworthy. Because of the geographical location, the activities were also apparent and obvious to everyone, radio communications were easily monitored, and the period coincided with a time of radical social change and an alteration in attitudes of the public to employers and their responsibilities. For all these reasons, the health of the offshore workers and their environment received a degree of public attention to which the industry had hitherto been unaccustomed, but which it has now come to accept as an inevitable part of its business.

And so it came about that the subject of offshore medicine was born. It is now in its adolescence and is rapidly maturing through the experience which has been gained in the challenging years from 1965. It impinges upon many people — the medics who are on the rigs, the GPs on shore, who provide the day-to-day cover and back-up service, the hospitals and community physicians, who bear the brunt of major accidents and incidents, the oil company doctors responsible for the organisation of it all and the Government medical services who ensure that standards are maintained, and the company management and administrators who have to pay for it.

The aim of this book is to bring together an account of the experience gained in the first decade or so of offshore medicine, to offer some standards and guide-lines to those who may be facing its problems for the first time, and to provide a source of information for those people, both doctors and others, who may be confronted with unique situations which they will not find described in any of the standard books on general, occupational or environmental medicine.

London, October 1981   R.A.F. Cox

Preface to the Second Edition

Since the first edition of this book was published in 1981, offshore exploration for and production of oil and gas have continued to expand in many parts of the world. Only now, with the recent decline in the price of oil, has activity begun to decrease. At the same time, offshore medicine has passed through its adolescence and has now reached its age of majority. There are many doctors involved in the provision of medical care for offshore communities around the globe and much of the experience gained has been utilised in providing medical services in other remote places such as the Antarctic.

Many agencies representing both employers and employees and groups such as the International Labour Organisation are taking an increasing interest in health and safety offshore while some government agencies have enacted legislation to improve standards. Fortunately, in general, standards are continuing to improve without the coercion of legislation. However, in some areas such as the design of hospitals on mobile drilling rigs, it is disappointing to observe that there has been almost no improvement in the design of their medical facilities and extensive modifications are required to brand new units before they can operate in some national waters, or for many responsible operators.

In the United Kingdom we have been waiting since January 1986 for the publication of the new Offshore Installation and Pipeline Works (First-Aid) Regulations. When they come into effect these Regulations will be a great step forward in raising the standards of medical care for workers in the United Kingdom sector of the North Sea. It had been hoped to include them in this book in their entirety, but debate, discussion and procrastination through the tripartite formulation process has caused such inordinate delays that this book must go to press before they are ready. It has, therefore, been necessary to summarise and paraphrase the proposed draft regulations in Appendix 8. It is not anticipated that the final version will differ significantly from the draft, but it does seem regrettable that such an important piece of legislation should be so delayed when the three parties have reached agreement concerning its content for many months.

Health and safety in the diving field has certainly continued to improve since the first edition was published, but there is now a real concern in the diving industry, among the general public and among the diving medical fraternity concerning the possible long-term effects of prolonged hyperbaric exposure. There is very little evidence that there are any permanent effects, but the only way to be sure and to allay anxiety is to put together an epidemiological survey of the medical data which are now being accumulated on divers' health as a result of their annual physical examinations. Unfortunately, the Health and Safety Executive, who are responsible for enforcing regulations concerning divers' health and their medical surveillance, have not accepted responsibility to investigate the long-term health effects and have, therefore, declined to set up any procedure for either generating or collecting the necessary data. Hopefully, the industry through one or more of the main centres where most divers are examined, will take up the initiative.

The offshore oil industry, as I leave it after twenty years of association with it, has changed markedly. Changed, I can certainly say, for the better; I hope that the present recession in the industry does not set back the great strides in health and safety to which I have been witness. There are still many improvements to be made and I hope that the second edition of this book will enable those managers, engineers, doctors, administrators, medics and others who are responsible, to maintain the momentum which has gathered since the first edition appeared.

London, August 1986   R.A.F. Cox

Acknowledgements

Numerous friends and colleagues have helped in many ways with the preparation of this book and I apologise unreservedly if I have forgotten to include any of their names. The following people and organisations come to mind for help of many kinds:

Ralph Spinks and Nick Wells for technical comments, John and Anne Bevan for help in many ways. Sue Journeaux for invaluable assistance, Ros Harris for help with the bibliography, Maurice Broomfield, Picture Coverage, and Oceaneering International for the use of photographs, Phillips Petroleum Company for the use of photographs and help in a hundred other ways, the UKOOA Medical Advisory Committee for many informal comments and the use of material originally prepared for it, the Diving Medical Advisory committee for the use of other documents, Dr. Trevor Robinson and Dr. Anthony Coleman for comments on certain aspects of dermatology and anaesthesia respectively, Miss M. Collins for secretarial assistance, the Dental Director General of the Royal Navy, the Controller of her Majesty's Stationery Office and last, but certainly not least, all my old colleagues at the North Sea Medical Centre, especially Dr. D.G. Watson and Mr. Steve Dick.

While much of the experience which has been incorporated into this book was gained in the course of my work with Phillips Petroleum, and for which I am very grateful, any opinions expressed are entirely my own and in no way reflect any actual or implied policies of the company.

Second Edition

Jawad Sa'd has reviewed and rewritten the first chapter and I am most grateful to him for this assistance. I also wish to thank Dr. Mark Harries and Dr. David Ziderman for their comments and advice on some aspects of the sections on resuscitation.

Contents

Contributors

I.K. Anderson, BA, BM, BChir, MRCGP, AFOM
Director and Physician to North Sea Medical Centre and Oilfield
Medical Services International Ltd., North Sea Medical Centre,
3 Lowestoft Road, Gorleston-on-Sea, Great Yarmouth, Norfolk.

I.M. Calder, MD
Honorary Senior Lecturer, Department of Morbid Anatomy, The
London Hospital Medical College, The London Hospital,
Whitechapel, London, E1 1BB

N. Chalk, FHCIMA, MRSH
Beech Farm, Upton, Nr. Acle, Norwich, NR13 6BP

R.A.F. Cox, MA, MB, BChir, FFOM
Chief Medical Officer, Central Electricity Board, Courtenay House,
18 Warwick Lane, London, EC4P 4BX

(formerly Medical Director, Phillips Petroleum Europe-Africa, The
Adelphie, John Adam Street, London, WC2 6BW)

A.J. Higginson, MA (CANTAB)
Legal Adviser, North Sea Sun Oil Company Limited, 90 Long Acre,
London, WC2E 9RA

P.B. James, MB, DIH, PhD, MFOM
Senior Lecturer in Occupational Medicine, University of Dundee,
Ninewells Hospital and Medical School, Dundee, DD1 9SY

J.N. Norman, MD, DSc, PhD, NSc, FRCS (Glas), FRCS (Edin),
FInst Biol, MInst Pet
Director, Centre for Offshore Health, Robert Gordon's Institute of
Technology, Kepplestone Mansion, Viewfield Road, Aberdeen,
AB9 2PF

D.J.G. Pyper, BDS
Consultant Dental Adviser, North Sea Medical Centre, 3 Lowestoft
Road, Gorleston-on-Sea, Great Yarmouth, Norfolk.

J. Sa'd
Senior Geologist, Phillips Petroleum Europe-Africa, The Adelphie,
John Adam Street, London, WC2N 6BW

Chapter 1

Introduction

J. Sa'd and R.A.F. Cox

Petroleum and natural gas are the remains of organic matter deposited and buried in the geological past. With time, temperature and bacterial action, a portion of the organic matter matures into hydrocarbons and migrates out of the source bed to porous and permeable reservoir rocks. The oil and gas generated will further migrate into more favourable geological conditions where they can be trapped and sealed. Conditions for hydrocarbon generation, migration and entrapment occur in the sedimentary basins of the world, both onshore and offshore.

Modern onshore oilwell drilling began in the 1860s, and offshore drilling began in the 1940s, when sunken barges and wooden-piled platforms were used. Oil has now been produced in water over 400 m deep, and the petroleum industry is currently investing money in the exploration of prospects lying under more than 2000 m water. The extraction of oil and gas from the earth may be divided into four phases:

1. Geological exploration
2. Exploratory drilling
3. Development
4. Production

Geological Exploration

Petroleum exploration aims towards finding hydrocarbons in commercial quantities. To reach this objective a series of data gathering and interpreting phases are usually followed.

Phase 1 is the stage of geological evaluation and reconnaissance geophysics. The objective of this stage is to throw light on the five factors that are critical to petroleum accumulation: (a) a mature source rock; (b) a migration path connecting source rock to reservoir rock; (c) a reservoir rock that is both porous and permeable; (d) a trap; and (e) an impermeable seal (Fig. 1.1).

Phase 2 is the stage of seismic survey. This phase may be associated with phase 1 in offshore exploration. During this stage more knowledge is gained of the depth configuration of potential traps and the character and volume of the sedimentary fill. The exploration geologist works closely with the geophysicist to integrate their data and establish a geological model. This will be followed by selecting the most promising prospect to be drilled. Phase 3 is the stage of exploration (or wildcat) drilling, which establishes a detailed sampling of the sediment character (reservoir, source and cap rock). At this stage even a dry hole is not necessarily a total failure. It

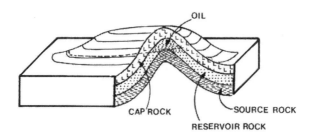

OIL ACCUMULATION IN AN ANTICLINAL STRUCTURE

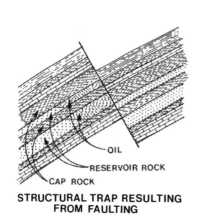

STRUCTURAL TRAP RESULTING FROM FAULTING

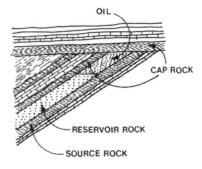

OIL ACCUMULATION UNDER AN UNCONFORMITY

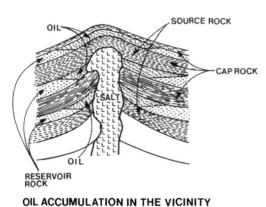

OIL ACCUMULATION IN THE VICINITY OF A PIERCEMENT TYPE SALT DOME

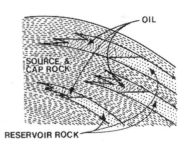

OIL ACCUMULATION IN SAND LENSES OF THE SAND BAR TYPE

Fig. 1.1. Hydrocarbon-bearing formations.

can supply a large amount of data which, if intelligently studied, may lead to the placement of new wildcat wells.

At all exploration stages a geological analogy is often used to compare the unexplored basin with other producing 'look-alike' basins which appear to have common geological characteristics. In offshore exploration the geologist may be aided by using side-scan sonar for mapping under water topographic-structural features, marine 'sniffer' surveys to record and evaluate gases leaking from the seafloor, and radiation surveys to detect seafloor surface patterns of uranium daughter elements concentrated above buried reservoirs.

The most diagnostic tools for the geophysicist are wildcat wells and seismic surveys. Aeromagnetic surveys, to reveal basement structures and basin configurations, provide a supplementary technique. Marine gravimeter surveys are less useful because the magnitude of the correction commonly exceeds the amplitudes of the anomalies.

Historically, marine seismic techniques were born and raised in the Gulf of Mexico, and the first seismic vessels were converted mud boats. Today, for international operations, and for high seas, the vessels are often of about 1000 tons gross, 70 m length, and fitted with a helicopter deck and two sophisticated navigation systems as the first and major problem in marine seismology is to know where the vessel is.

The vessel towing strings of hydrophones through the water discharges an energy source at regular intervals to provide the sound transient. The sound is reflected from interfaces between rocks of different acoustical conductivity and the reflected sound waves are sensed by the hydrophones and recorded (Fig. 1.2). By combining computer manipulation of these data and geological interpretation, a contour map of the structure (or feature) promising hydrocarbon accumulation can be obtained.

Assessing prospectivity in producing regions is wholly different from that in frontier regions. In the former, the presence of oil is known, and the question is whether enough undrilled prospects remain between, beyond, above and especially below known fields in order to justify further exploration. Much well data is usually available, and the main geological effort is geared towards answering questions of geological detail before planning further geophysical surveys.

If seismic surveying shows promising structures, a field office will be organised in preparation for exploratory drilling. The facilities required include office space, warehousing, a helipad, and docks. In addition, local workers must be hired, materials procured, and plans made for medical evacuation of offshore personnel.

Service companies (subcontractors) will also be contracted at this time. The oil company that is drilling or developing a field finances, engineers and organises the project, but nearly all the work is done by service company personnel. Some of these companies are:

Drilling

1. Drilling contractors
2. Drilling-mud service
3. Drilling data (mud) loggers
4. Cementing and stimulation services
5. Electronic logging
6. Divers
7. Drilling stem test services

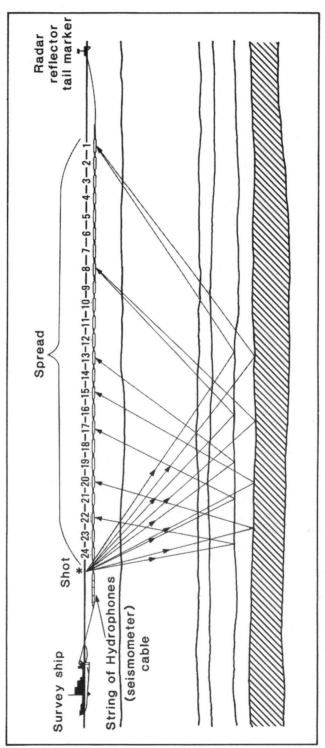

Fig. 1.2.   A diagram illustrating the principles of reflective seismology.

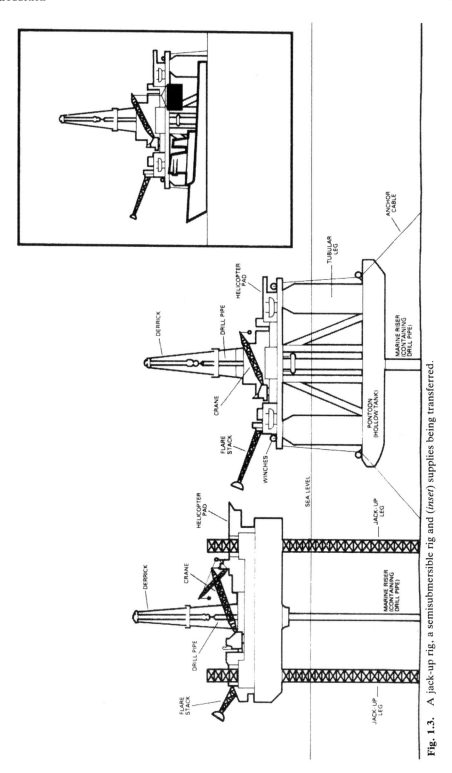

Fig. 1.3. A jack-up rig, a semisubmersible rig and (*inset*) supplies being transferred.

8. Helicopter operators
9. Tug-, supply-, stand-by- and workboat operators
10. Specialised tool and equipment suppliers and services

Development

1. Platform designers
2. Platform constructors
3. Derrick barge operators
4. Pipelay barge operators
5. Equipment suppliers

Drilling Rigs

The equipment necessary to drill a well is known collectively as a *rig*: The most important components of the rig are:

1. The *drillstring*, an assembly of drillpipe, the drillbit, and miscellaneous tools which are rotated to drill the hole
2. The *rotary table* which rotates the drillstring
3. The *draw-works*, large winches that raise and lower the drillstring
4. The *mud circulation system*, which recovers, filters and reinjects the *drilling mud*
5. The *derrick*, the tower that supports the weight of the drillstring

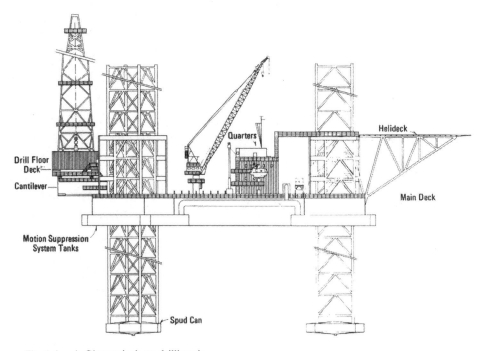

Fig. 1.4. A Glomar jack-up drilling rig.

6. The navigation that allows the rig to be positioned precisely over the selected drilling location.

Offshore rigs may be mounted on a *platform* (a fixed structure) for development drilling, but must be mobile for exploratory drilling. Mobile rigs are usually classified by their means of support (Fig. 1.3):

Bottom-supported

1. *Barges*, which are flooded and sink to the bottom
2. *Submersibles*, bottom-resting but with the rig floor several metres above the water line to provide protection from waves
3. *Jack-ups*, which lift themselves out of the water on legs (Fig. 1.4)

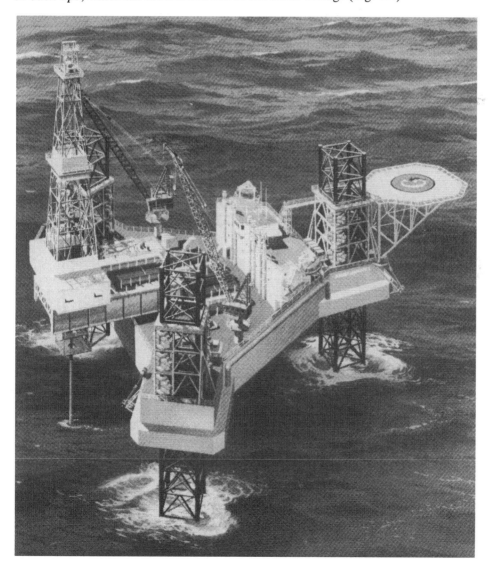

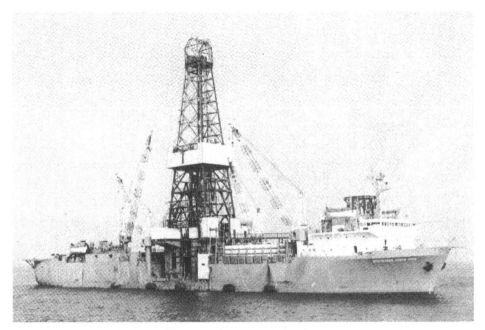

Fig. 1.5.   The drill ship Discoverer Seven Seas.

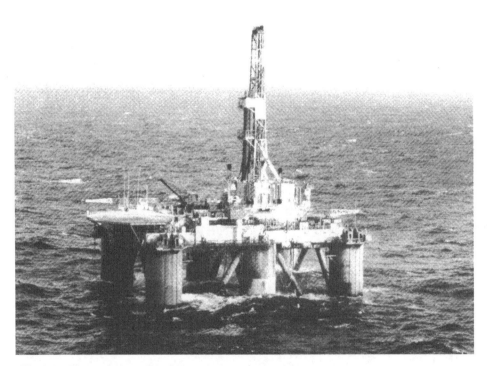

Fig. 1.6.   The semisubmersible drilling rig Western Pacesetter.

Floating

1. *Barges*, which are towed and anchored by tugs
2. *Drillships*, which are self-propelled (Fig. 1.5)
3. *Semisubmersibles*, whose equipment is mounted out of the reach of waves on legs supported by ballasted pontoons (Fig. 1.6)

Bottom-supported units are economically preferable in water less than 100 m deep and floating vessels in deeper water. Drillships and barges are more easily moved and are common in remote locations.

A floating drilling rig must obviously be kept stationary over the hole. In *dynamic positioning*, a computer-controlled propulsion system continuously holds the vessel over the hole. An older and more common approach is the use of anchors, typically eight in number, which are set with the help of a supply boat that carries or tows the anchors into position.

Exploratory Drilling

At any given time there may be 50–100 men present on a typical offshore drilling rig. The *company man* (officially, the drilling superintendent or drilling engineer) is often the only employee representing the oil company that is drilling the well (a company geologist is often present on location while drilling the objective horizons), and is in charge of the operation under normal conditions. Working closely with him is the *toolpusher*, who is the drilling contractor's manager. Subordinate to the toolpusher are two *drillers*, alternating on 12-h shifts, who operate the draw-works controls and direct three to five *roughnecks* working on the rig floor and in the derrick. These men are normally assisted in drilling operations by specialists representing various service companies: mud engineers, cementing crews, casing crews, logging crews, etc. Many nationalities will be represented on the mobile drilling rig. Although the people engaged in drilling must speak a common language (usually English), the ship's crew and general labourers may speak only their native languages. English is usually spoken by their *pusher* (boss). In a parallel organisation are the ship's crew, caterers, mechanics, *roustabouts* (general labourers not directly involved in drilling), etc.

A primary consideration during the drilling of a well is containment of the pressurised formations encountered beneath the surface of the earth. *Normal pressure* at a given depth is the pressure exerted by a column of saltwater of equivalent height, but abnormal pressures up to twice this amount can be found (thus, care must be taken when drilling exploratory wells in a new area). The borehole is kept filled at all times with *drilling mud* of density great enough to balance the normal or abnormal pressures; if this is not done a *blowout* (uncontrolled discharge of well fluids or gases) could result.

Drilling mud, despite its name, is a sophisticated and expensive chemical mixture that has several functions in addition to pressure control; cooling and lubricating the bit, suspending and removing rock cuttings, and supporting the borehole wall. Its density, flow characteristics, solids content, and rate of water loss (i.e. leakage into permeable formations) are constantly monitored by a *mud engineer*. The mud circulates down the drillstring, up the drillstring borehole annulus, through the *shale-shaker screens* (for the removal of rock cuttings), and back into the mudpumps. Drilling mud normally contains *water* (fresh or salt) as the continuous phase, although oil can be used, *weighting materials* (particles of suspended solids), *viscosifiers* (usually clays), and *water-loss control agents* (polymeric compounds) as well as rock cuttings and formation fluids. In addition, several special-purpose additives may be used (some of them proprietary): dispersants (of the suspended clays), oil, inhibitors (of rock reactions), acids or bases, foam suppressants, corrosion inhibitors, and loss circulation materials (macroscopic particles which prevent the loss of whole mud to permeable formations).

After the rig is set on location, the first step in drilling a well is to set structural pipe in the seabed (typically 100 m deep). Then a drillbit and *collars* (heavy-duty drillpipe) are lowered into the structural pipe, and a hexagonal length of drillpipe (the *kelly*) at the top of the drillstring is turned by the rotary table. *'Clear' water* is used for drilling mud and is not returned to the rig. When 30 ft of hole has been drilled, the drillstring is suspended by *slips* in the rig floor while the kelly is unscrewed and a new *joint* of pipe is inserted into the string.

Periodically during drilling it is necessary to *trip out*, or remove the drillstring, in order to change the bit or perform repairs. This means rapid strenuous work for the *roughnecks* (Fig. 1.7), as three joints (a *stand*) of pipe are pulled at a time and racked vertically by a *derrickman* situated near the top of the derrick. Mud must be constantly added to the hole to replace the pipe volume. Drilling is conducted 24 h per day in all weather except the most severe storms.

After drilling to a certain depth (of the order of 500 m below *mud line*) it is

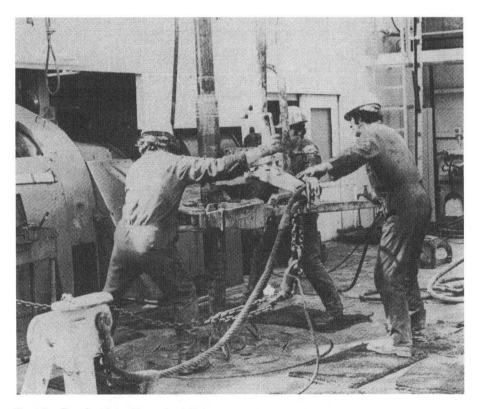

Fig. 1.7. Roughneck 'making up' a drillpipe connection with tongs.

necessary to run *casing*, large-diameter pipe lowered into the hole and cemented in place. Casing helps prevent loss of drilling mud and underground blowouts (which occur when the difference in pressure between two zones is less than the difference in the hydrostatic head of the mud column). Two to four strings of casing are normally run, telescope fashion, to allow changes in mud weight and to decrease the risk resulting from having large amounts of naked rock wall exposed at the same time. Before running casing through prospective hydrocarbon zones, the well is *logged* with electronic instruments lowered on a *wireline* able to detect hydrocarbons and give information about rock properties.

Casing requires heavier-duty equipment and often special crews of roughnecks. Once run into the hole it is supported by the surface pipe and cemented into place. More specialists and equipment are required for cementing, which is done by pumping a cement and water mixture down the casing, followed by water and drilling mud that push the cement into the casing borehole annulus. This requires careful planning and execution, as high pressures are necessary to 'U-tube' the dense cement up the annulus, and the cement will solidify in a few hours whether it is in place or not.

After the first string of casing has been cemented into place the *blowout preventers* (BOPs) are installed. These are a collection of very large valves that can close off the borehole even with drillpipe in place. When drilling from a bottom-supported or platform-mounted rig, the first casing string usually extends upwards to the rig (i.e. above the surface of the water) and the BOPs are mounted on top. On a floating rig the BOPs are set at seafloor level and a *marine riser* pipe connects the BOPs to the rig. Once the BOPs (and riser if necessary) have been connected, drilling mud can be circulated into the hole and recovered at the surface.

After each string of casing is run, drilling is continued with a smaller bit until total depth has been reached. A potential hydrocarbon zone can then be chosen from the logs and entered with a *perforating gun*. The perforating gun is lowered on a wireline and uses small, accurately positioned charges to blast holes through the casing and cement.

At this point an exploratory well is ready to be tested. Drillpipe with a special assembly of tools is lowered into the hole and partially filled with water from above. One of the tools, a *packer*, expands around the outside of the string to seal against the inside of the casing. A valve below the packer is opened, and allows formation pressure from the perforations to enter the drillstring and unload the watercushion; the well should flow without assistance because the weight of the hydrocarbon column in the drillstring is less than the normal (i.e. saltwater column) pressure in the formation. In underpressured formations pumping or other methods of artificial lifting will be needed.

If the well does not flow sufficiently, *stimulation* may be attempted to reduce flow restriction in the rock around the borehole. *Acidisation* will dissolve mud impurities and carbonaceous rocks. *Fracturing* will open larger flow channels in the rock; this can be done by pumping a fluid into the formation at high rates and pressures followed by a proppant to hold the artificial crevices open.

After the zone's deliverability has been measured, it will be *squeezed off* by pumping cement into the perforations and another zone can be tested. When all the zones have been squeezed off, an exploratory well will usually be permanently abandoned even if productive. This is due to damage after testing and squeezing and the difficulty of tying the well into production facilities brought in at a later date.

Development

After the exploratory and delineation or confirmation wells have been drilled and tested, a commercial find will be developed for long-term production. This requires:

1. Installation of a platform with process equipment
2. Drilling of development wells
3. Provision for the transportation of the produced oil and/or gas

Development is conducted under the supervision of an on-site oil company representative.

The *fixed-pile platform* (Fig. 1.8) is the oldest and most common offshore structure. The *jacket* (the legs and their cross braces) is constructed in an onshore yard and barged or towed floating to the site. The jacket is then set into position on the

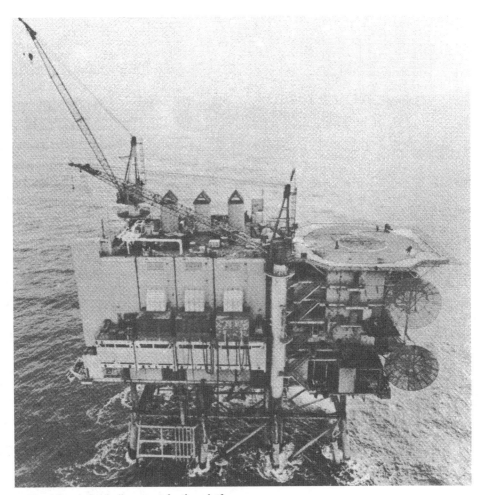

Fig. 1.8.   A fixed-pile gas production platform.

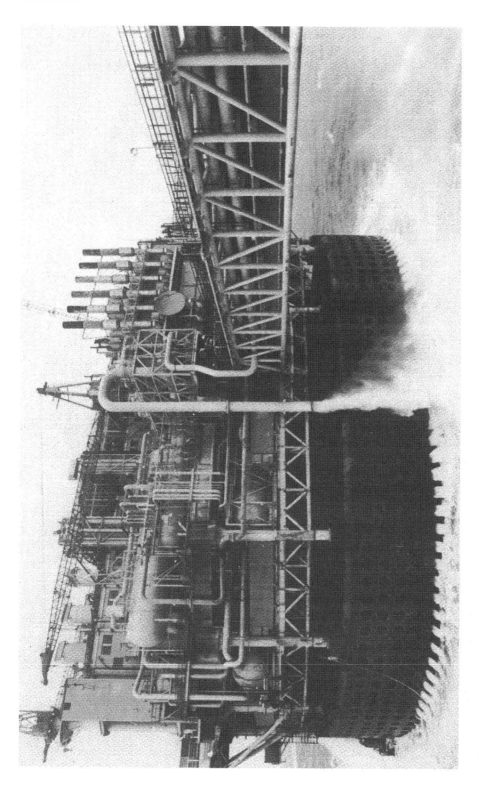

Fig. 1.9. A production complex. In the centre is a concrete gravity structure for the storage of oil and production equipment.

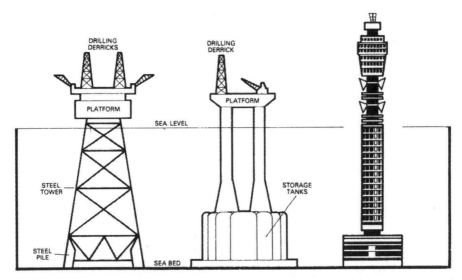

Fig. 1.10. A fixed-pile platform and a gravity platform compared with the Telecom Tower, London.

seafloor and piles are driven down through the legs to hold it in place. *Derrick barges* (crane-bearing vessels) lift the *decks*, equipment modules, crew quarters, rig, etc. into place. The decks are typically 50 ft or more above the mean water line, to place them out of the reach of waves generated by storms.

Another type of platform less commonly used is the *gravity structure* (Fig. 1.9), which is held in place only by its weight. This approach may allow the entire platform, including equipment modules, etc. to be assembled onshore. While piled platforms are of steel construction, gravity platforms may be steel, concrete, or a combination of the two (Fig. 1.10). The next generation of platforms will include, for deep water, buoyant platforms held in place by *tension legs* (Fig. 1.11) and compliant *guyed towers*.

There are several alternatives to the most common course of setting a production platform, followed by drilling the development wells. The wells may be *pre-drilled* with a mobile rig through a seafloor *template* before the platform is constructed and set, giving earlier production (Fig. 1.12). A platform design which allows the drilling of development wells with a mobile rig may be used to avoid the purchase of a drilling rig. In a third scheme, the production platform is fed by one or more nearby *well-protector platforms* (carrying wellheads but no production facilities) or by *subsea-completed* wells (with their wellheads either in groups or at individual sites on the seafloor).

Setting a platform or jacket requires calm water and close coordination. A small barge-carried structure may be lifted from the cargo barge with a crane, but larger ones must be pulled off by tugs or launched from specially equipped barges. The structure's descent can be controlled to a certain extent by selective flooding, and it can be guided into position by a crane barge. After the platform and its modules have been set, there are normally several months of hook-up and commissioning work before it is ready for production.

The platform's position and structural integrity will be checked by divers. Divers are first present offshore in support of exploratory drilling, and return to the field through the development and production phases.

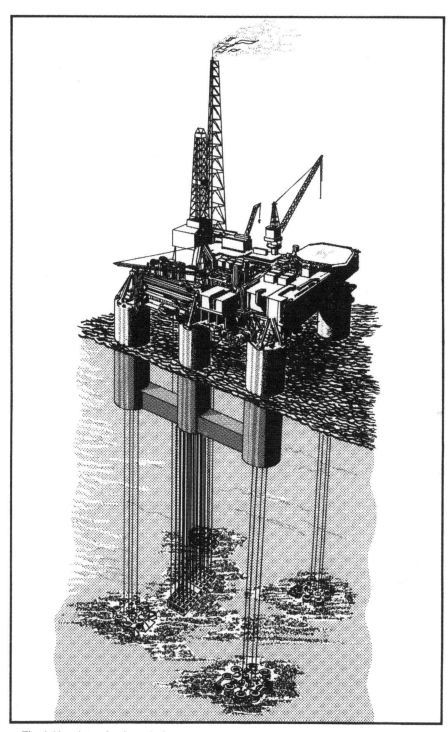

Fig. 1.11. A tension legs platform.

Installation in the Field   Into Production

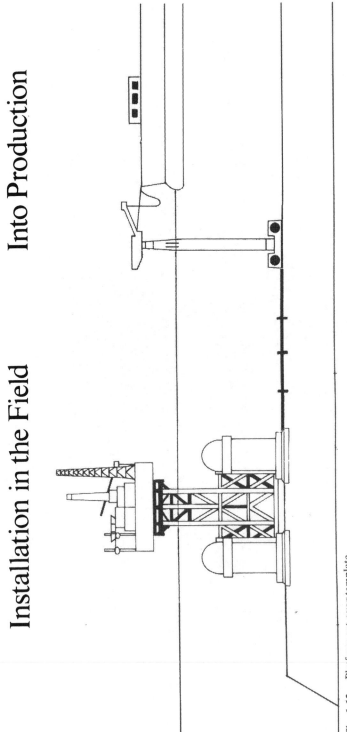

Fig. 1.12.   Platform set over template.

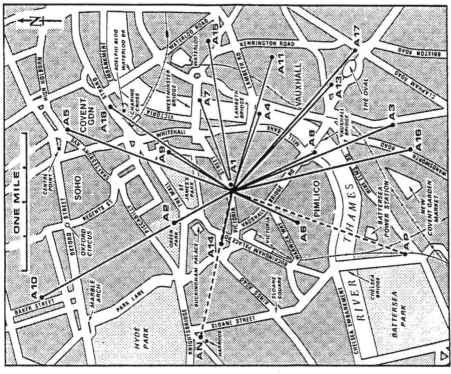

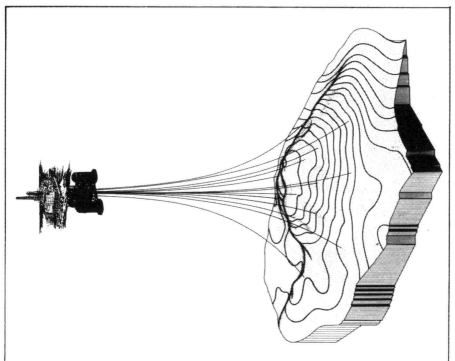

Fig. 1.13. Deviated wells in Maureen Field. The map shows the bottom hole locations supposing the platform to be located in Victoria Street, London.

The drilling of development wells is fundamentally the same as the drilling of exploratory wells. After drilling straight down for a few hundred metres, the well may be *deviated* (curved outwards) to reach a distant target; this allows as many as 60 wells to be drilled from a single platform (Fig. 1.13). Rather than testing with drillpipe as described earlier, the well is completed with *tubing* (2–5 in. diameter pipe) for permanent production and is equipped with safety shutdown devices. A wellhead and *christmas tree* (a cluster of valves) is mounted on top of the well and the well fluids can then be directed into the production system.

Pipelines are usually laid to transmit the produced fluid to shore. On board a *pipelaying barge* (Fig. 1.14), a team of welders continuously welds together lengths of pipe, radiographs them, coats them and passes them off the stern of the barge (Fig. 1.15). The barge is tended by supply boats carrying pipe, and tugboats that move its anchors forward one at a time. After the pipe is laid on the seafloor, another barge will waterblast a trench into which the pipe falls and is buried by natural backfill. Pipelines may also be laid by towing them from an assembly point onshore, or by unreeling the completed line from spools. Connection of the pipeline to the platform often requires divers or remote-controlled equipment.

In remote locations it may not be economically feasible to construct a pipeline to shore. In this situation, a short pipeline connects the platform to a *mooring buoy* from which a tanker can load oil (Fig. 1.16). Produced gas must be *flared* (burned) or reinjected into the reservoir.

Production

When development drilling is finished and production begins, the platform becomes the charge of the *operator* (or *production superintendent*). He is responsible for daily maintenance, the enforcement of safety rules, supervising contract workers, etc. The operator has an assistant who can deputise for him. Specialists are also intermittently present during production operations: mechanics, electricians, instrument men, etc. Most men on offshore production platforms (Figs. 1.17 and 1.18) work a nominal 12 h per day with alternating weeks of work and rest. The language problem is not as great as in the drilling and development phases because fewer men and organisations are involved.

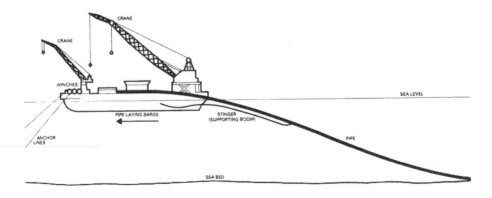

Fig. 1.14. Diagram of a pipelay barge at work.

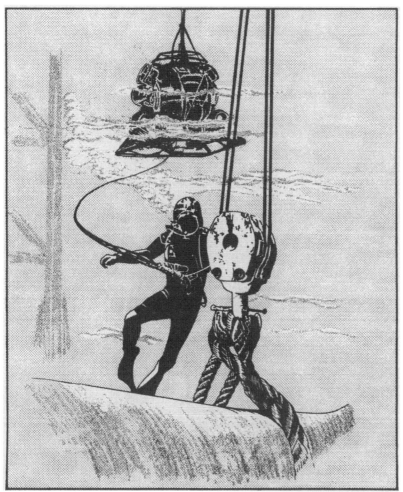

Fig. 1.15.   A pipelay diver at work.

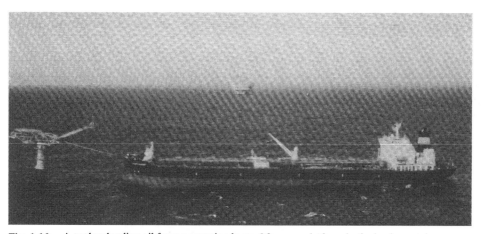

Fig. 1.16.   A tanker loading oil from a mooring buoy. Maureen platform in the background.

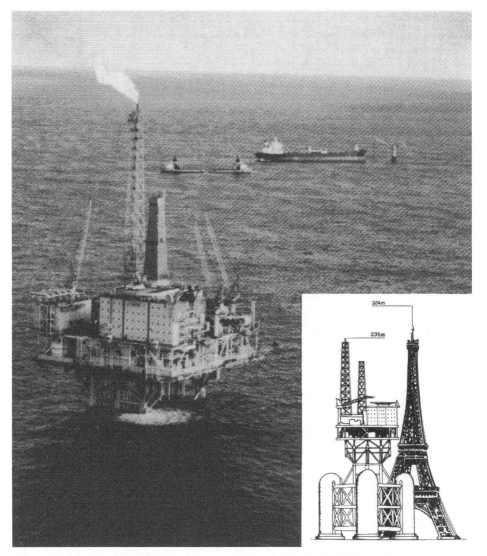

Fig. 1.17. Maureen production platform compare (*inset*) with the Eiffel Tower, Paris.

The produced fluids from each well flow through a *choke* for pressure equalisation and then into the production system, which normally operates at various pressures between 1000 and 100 psi. The oil, gas and water phases are separated and purified; the oil is pumped into a pipeline, the gas is flared or compressed and pipelined, and the water is discharged overboard.

All platforms have an *emergency shutdown system* (ESD). The ESD system is a network of pressure, temperature, flow and chemical composition sensors coupled to pneumatically operated *motor-valves* and switches throughout the production system. When an abnormal situation is detected, the ESD automatically shuts down

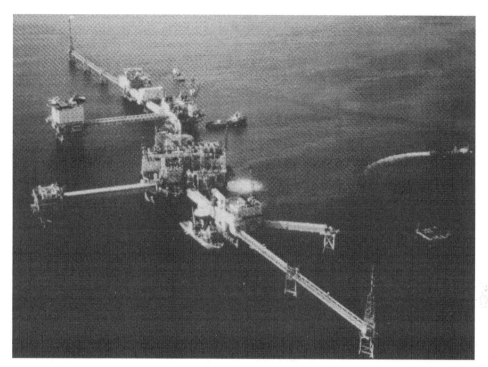

Fig. 1.18.   Production complex, Ekofisk Centre. The distance between the two flare stacks is nearly 1 km.

and isolates all or part of the platform's equipment, including below-mud-line safety valves in the wells.

Other major equipment and systems found on a production platform may include generators, firewater pumps, cranes, a helipad, living quarters, and the instrument-air supply system. Some platforms have potable water makers, sewage systems, and oil storage capacity. More uncommon are platform-mounted *gas plants* which condense the liquid vapours in the natural gas to form *natural gas liquids*. Most platforms have fireproof escape boats.

During the field's producing life, usually 20 years or more, the producing well will require several *workovers* (downhole repairs). This often involves using a rig to replace tubing, squeeze off a depleted zone and re-perforate, etc. and is similar to a small-scale drilling operation. Whenever drilling or workover operations are conducted simultaneously with production, the platform operator is responsible for safety and has the authority to halt either or both activities.

As fluid is produced from the reservoir, the pressure in that reservoir normally declines and production rates decrease. To counteract this, *artificial lift* may be employed, either *pumping* or *gas lift* (bubbling gas through the tubing to lighten the fluid column). *Pressure maintenance* may be attempted by injecting gas or water into the reservoir.

At the end of the field's life, most governments require that the wells be plugged permanently and the platforms removed.

Communications and Transport

Rig communications are most often provided by a radio link to a shore base which is manned 24 h per day. Platform communications may be by radio, microwave or telephone cable.

Personnel and light goods are normally transported by helicopters carrying 3–44 passengers per trip. Night and rough weather flights can be arranged if necessary and, in emergencies, governmental organisations such as the US Coast Guard and the British Royal Air Force may provide specialised rescue aircraft.

A variety of boats and ships are used in offshore operations:

1. *Tankers* are occasionally seen when pipelines are not feasible.
2. *Drilling tenders* may be moored alongside a rig, carrying some of its equipment.
3. *Tugboats* are used to move mobile rigs, derrick barges, etc.
4. *Anchor-handling boats* are fitted with winches and other gear.
5. *Supply boats*, (Fig. 1.19) the 'workhorses' of the industry, are typically 50 m long and designed with open deck space for large items; they may also be equipped to serve as tugs, anchor-handlers, etc. *Workboats* and *crewboats* are smaller utility vessels.
6. Special-purpose boats are available for oilspill cleanup, firefighting, etc.

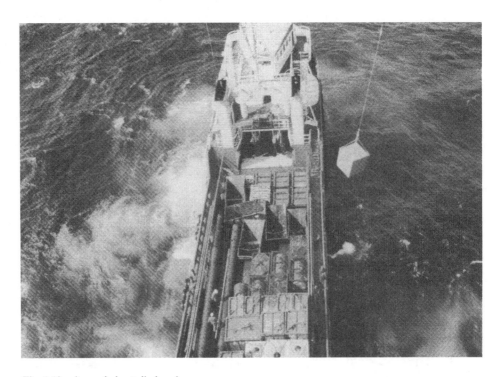

Fig. 1.19   A supply boat discharging cargo.

Hazards

Although the bulk of reported injuries offshore result from mishandling heavy equipment, slipping, and other common industrial accidents, offshore work provides additional hazards:

1. *Harsh Environments.* These range from ice islands to tropical swamps. Storms on the open sea are an unavoidable danger.
2. *Remote Locations.* Operations may be conducted in areas several hours distant by air from the nearest hospital and medical evacuations are subject to the weather.
3. *Blowouts and Well Fires.* Fires have been known to melt platforms down to the water line.
4. *Toxic and Flammable Chemicals.* In addition to artificial materials, offshore workers may be exposed to hydrogen sulphide in some natural gases.

Costs of Offshore Operations

Geological exploration is relatively inexpensive, costing only a few hundreds of thousands of U.S.\$ per discovery. Exploratory drilling has often cost up to U.S.\$150 000 per day, with a current average of U.S.\$10 million per well. Once a field is discovered, an average of 10–15 wells are needed to produce the field. Development is the most expensive phase; developing a large field with more than one platform may require an investment of billions of dollars. The operating costs of a producing field may reach U.S.\$250 000 per day. Prices vary widely according to location and environment.

Implications for the Doctor

The offshore oil industry is one of frenetic activity and enormous costs. Any delay means the loss of a lot of money, which is why it may sometimes be cheaper to charter a jet to fly the Atlantic with a small piece of vital equipment or a few tons of special sand, or, equally, why pressure may be put upon an attending physician to return a particular expert back to work with the minimum of delay. For the same reason it may be cheaper to fly a doctor to a rig to attend a vital member of the crew at a critical time than to send the crew member ashore and hold up the drilling or construction programme.

Planning in the offshore industry is often difficult because of unpredictable factors such as weather, unexpected drilling problems, equipment delays or changes in government policy, and so everyone in the industry is accustomed to thinking and acting with great urgency — as the saying goes 'we want it yesterday'.

The doctor who is going to provide a service to this industry must be prepared to accept this sort of urgency about everything — an urgency which has nothing to do with medical priorities. He must be prepared to respond with equal alacrity when requested and he must be prepared to accept these apparently insatiable demands which the industry may put upon him. But, in return, it will not expect him to give his services without proper reward.

Finally, since the oil industry is an international one, it is inevitable that the doctor who becomes involved with it will find himself working with a very wide horizon, and he is likely to have to travel abroad himself on occasions.

The cost of such medical care is fractionally small compared with the overall cost of the operations, and the cost of failure of medical care may be extremely expensive. Though to the doctor it may be inconvenient and annoying to be asked to attend a medically non-urgent casualty in the middle of the night, to the company the doctor's decision on the man's fitness to continue work or not may mean several thousand pounds in charter fees for supply boats or helicopters. In the frantic rush to work while nature allows, no delay is acceptable and the doctor's role in avoiding delays is vital.

Incidence of Major Mishaps

Clemmer and Diem (1985) reviewed the major mishaps to mobile offshore drilling units in the period 1955–1981. They found that the frequency has increased in recent years though the trend in relation to the size of the fleet has remained stable in spite of improvement of rig designs by industry classification societies and increasing regulation by government agencies. They found a higher rate of mishaps among jack-up rigs and a total of 344 deaths secondary to major incidents. This figure does not include fatalities arising from routine industrial operations.

Bibliography

British Medical Association (1975) The medical implications of oil-related industry. BMA, London
Clemmer DI, Diem JE (1985) Major mishaps among mobile offshore drilling units, 1955–1981. Time trends and fatalities. Int J Epidemiol 14(1)
Cox, RAF (1970) Medical services to offshore drilling. Injury 1(3)
Cumming RP, Taylor W (1973) Aspects of health in oil development. The Shetland Times Ltd

Chapter 2

Legal Aspects of Safety, Health and Welfare on the United Kingdom Continental Shelf*

A.J. Higginson

In this chapter it is proposed to consider the laws relating to safety, health and welfare on the continental shelf of the United Kingdom. The particular legislation is considered briefly later, as well as liability insurance for employers. However, before reviewing such legislation, and to appreciate its evolution, it is important to note how international law has come to recognise the jurisdictional claims of coastal states over the waters of their continental shelf, long regarded as the high seas, in what is now known as the continental shelf doctrine.

The Continental Shelf Doctrine

Territorial Waters, Contiguous Zones and Continental Shelves

The extent of a country's territorial waters, and the rights exercisable over it, have been argued endlessly since Roman law branded the sea as *res communis*. However, the United Kingdom has for a long time claimed rights over its territorial waters [1], and it has long been recognised that though any foreign vessel has a right of innocent passage, such vessel must comply with all applicable laws and regulations, including those relating to health, and the Territorial Waters Jurisdiction Act 1878 vested in the Admiralty Court jurisdiction over any offence committed in territorial waters.

With regard to the extent of territorial waters, apart from some Latin American countries, most countries have claimed between 3 and 12 miles. The Territorial Waters Jurisdiction Act 1878 recognised 3 miles, but the United Kingdom has fixed no limit, it being recognised that it might change as international custom and practice change [2]. Until recently, the most important issue with regard to territorial waters was the preservation of exclusive fishing rights by a country, and in the great majority of countries (including the United Kingdom) fishing limits are now set at 12 miles. In addition, during the nineteenth century it became generally recognised that a country's police and revenue jurisdiction extended beyond its territorial waters for a distance of 9 miles, and this area became known as the contiguous zone. This

---

*Legal References are listed at the end of this chapter.

jurisdictional extension was recognised by the 1958 Geneva Convention on the Territorial Sea and the Contiguous Zone [3], which provided that

the coastal state may exercise the control necessary to:
a) Prevent infringement of its . . . sanitary regulations within its territory or territorial sea.
b) Punish infringement of the above regulations committed within its territory or territorial sea [4].

It also limited the contiguous zone to a distance of 12 miles from the baseline from which the territorial sea is measured [5].

However, the international legal uncertainty of the extent of the juridical character of territorial seas was further complicated by the continental shelf doctrine. A common feature of maritime countries in the world is the presence of a shelf adjacent to their coastlines. This shelf is formed by the gradual decline in the seabed from the shoreline to a water depth of approximately 200 m, and the sudden, very steep, decline in the seabed thereafter. This phenomenon is now known as the 'continental shelf', though in the North Sea this feature is evidenced not by any shelf, but by the fact that the whole North Sea forms a shallow basin. As technology developed, maritime countries acquired an ability to explore and exploit the natural resources of their adjoining continental shelves, but the legality of such exploration was uncertain. In 1945, regulation of oil drilling operations in the Gulf of Mexico outside the territorial waters of the United States being required, the Truman Proclamation was issued, claiming rights for the United States in its continental shelf, and this proclamation led to similar claims by other countries.

The 1958 Geneva Convention on the Continental Shelf [6] provided that 'the Coastal State exercises over the continental shelf sovereign rights for the purposes of exploring it and exploiting its natural resources' [7]. The Convention defined the term 'continental shelf' as

the seabed and subsoil of the submarine areas adjacent to the coast but outside the territorial sea, to a depth of 200 metres or, beyond the limit, to where the superjacent waters admits of the exploration of the natural resources of the said areas.

and similar submarine areas adjacent to coasts of islands [8].

The extension of sovereign rights and the continental shelf doctrine are now accepted as customary international law, notwithstanding that seaward of territorial waters has long been regarded as the high seas [9] where the seas are 'free' [10] and over which no state may exercise control. Articles 4 and 5 of the Geneva Convention on the Continental Shelf [11] allow a country to establish offshore installations on its continental shelf in order to explore and exploit the natural resources, provided the traditional 'high seas' rights of other nations to lay cables and pipelines and to fish and navigate are not unjustifiably interfered with. However, in practice, maritime countries have found no difficulty in extending their jurisdiction, and resultant control, over their continental shelves, and the shelf in the North Sea is recognised as a natural prolongation of land over which the maritime state exercises sovereignty, and sovereign rights over it may simply be declared [12].

The United Kingdom Continental Shelf

In 1964, the Continental Shelf Act was passed in order to make provision for the exploration and exploitation of the continental shelf and 'give effect to certain provisions of the Convention on the High Seas' [13]. The Act simply vested in Her

Majesty 'any rights exercisable by the United Kingdom outside territorial waters with respect to the sea bed and subsoil and their natural resources' (except coal) [14]. The Act did not specify the 'rights', it being implicit that such 'rights' are those recognised by international law.

In relation to any petroleum [15], the Act provided that the licensing arrangements applicable onshore in Great Britain would be extended offshore [16], and should include provision for 'the safety, health and welfare of persons employed on operations undertaken under the authority of any Licence [17]'. The Act further provided [18] that any area within which the 'rights' are exercisable would be so designated from time to time by Her Majesty, and today areas surrounding all of the United Kingdom have been 'designated', extending in places to over 400 miles from the coastline and in water depths exceeding 1000 ft [19].

Section 3 of the Act provides that any 'act or omission which takes place on, or under or above an installation in a designated area' and within 500 m of such an installation shall, if such act or omission is an offence under the law of part of the United Kingdom, be similarly treated as such an offence. Thus Section 3 extended to offshore installations the civil and criminal laws of the United Kingdom, and The Continental Shelf (Jurisdiction) Order 1968 [20] applies the laws of and grants jurisdiction to England, Scotland and Northern Ireland in respect of acts or omissions occurring in the English, Scottish or Northern Irish areas of the continental shelf. In respect of the statutory laws of the United Kingdom, they will not apply to the territorial waters and the United Kingdom continental shelf unless expressly so provided in the relevant statute or by Order in Council.

It should be noted that the Oil and Gas (Enterprise) Act 1982 provides for the repeal and reenactment with amendments of Section 3 of the Continental Shelf Act 1964, but to date no commencement order has been made bringing the relevant provisions of the 1982 Act into effect [21].

Safety, Health and Welfare Legislation on the United Kingdom Continental Shelf [22]

As already mentioned, the Continental Shelf Act 1964 provided that the rights to explore and exploit petroleum on the continental shelf would be contained in and granted by a statutory licence [23]. The Model Clauses for production licences in seaward areas [24] provide that the

> Licensee shall comply with any instructions from time to time given by the Minister [25] in writing for securing the safety, health and welfare of persons employed in or about the licensed area [26].

Otherwise the production licence makes no express provision for safety, health and welfare on offshore installations, and safety, health and welfare legislation is to be found in the statutes and the regulations discussed below.

It is usual to have more than one person licensed in respect of an offshore area although, notwithstanding the plurality of licensees, each is both jointly and severally liable [26]. Further, one of the licensees, with the prior written approval of the 'Minister' [27], will have to act as operator responsible for organising or supervising operations [28] and the operator licensee will be concerned to ensure that all applicable safety, health and welfare legislation is observed.

Offshore Installations and Pipelines

The Mineral Workings (Offshore Installations) Act 1971 (the '1971 Act')

The 1971 Act applies to any of the specified activities which are carried on from any installation maintained in the water, or on the foreshore or other land intermittently covered with water, and which is not connected with dry land by a permanent structure providing access at all times and for all purposes [29]. The specified activities are: exploitation or exploration of mineral resources; storage or recovery of gas; conveyance of things by pipeline; and the provision of accommodation for persons working in the aforementioned activities [30].

The 1971 Act places the responsibility of ensuring that all offshore installations comply with regulations issued pursuant to the Act with the owner of the installation, the licensees and the installation manager [31]. However, the licensees are not responsible in respect of installations other than those maintained or established for underwater exploitation or exploration, nor for an installation comprising only apparatus associated with a pipeline (such as a booster station), unless the licensee has a right to exploit mineral resources in the area of such installations [32]. The installation manager is appointed by the owner of the installation and must be 'a person who, and to the best of the knowledge and belief of the owner, has the skill and competence for the appointment', and particulars of the appointee must be notified by the owner to the Secretary of State [33].

The installation manager has a statutory duty to be ever present on the installation, and to be responsible for

> matters affecting safety, health or welfare or, where connected with safety, health or welfare, the maintenance of order and discipline, and for the discharge of that responsibility shall exercise authority over all persons in or about the installation [34].

The manager has wide powers, including the right to put a person ashore [35], and to take such measures as are necessary or expedient in 'an emergency or apprehended emergency endangering the seaworthiness or stability of the installation or otherwise involving a risk of death or serious personal injury' [36]. For example, such wide powers could be used to deal with a person suffering from a mental disorder offshore, where the Mental Health Act 1959 does not apply. Further, any such measures taken by the installation manager shall not be prohibited or restricted by any regulation or condition having effect by virtue of the 1971 Act [36]. However, breach by any person of his statutory duty is actionable in so far as the breach causes personal injury [37], and may lead to criminal prosecution if an offence, as created by any regulations issued pursuant to the 1971 Act, is committed [38]. Any prosecution in respect of an offence may be only instigated by the Secretary of State or the Director of Public Prosecutions [39], and if committed by a body corporate with the consent and connivance of its director, manager or other officer, the latter, as well as the body corporate, may be held guilty of the offence [40].

Section 6 of the 1971 Act empowers the Secretary of State to make regulations for:

The safety, health and welfare of persons on offshore installations

The safety of such installations

The prevention of accidents on or near them

The schedule to the Act details the subject matter to be covered by such regulations, including the appointment of inspectors with powers to obtain access to an installation, and to hold public inquiries into any casualties or other accidents involving loss of life or danger to life. There have been numerous regulations issued pursuant to Section 6 [41], but the more important with regard to the subject matter discussed here are:

1. The Offshore Installations (Operational Safety, Health and Welfare) Regulations 1976
2. The Offshore Installations (Emergency Procedure) Regulations 1976
3. The offshore Installations (Inspectors and Casualties) Regulations 1973
4. The Diving Operations at Work Regulations 1981

The application clauses of the Regulations referred to in 1 and 2 above and the Offshore Installations (Life-Saving Appliances) Regulations 1977 [41] and the Offshore Installations (Fire Fighting Equipment) Regulations 1978 [41] have been amended so that the Regulations apply to any offshore installation (other than a dredging installation registered as a vessel) which is maintained in controlled waters for the carrying on of activities referred to in Section 1 of the 1971 Act as amended [42].

The Offshore Installations (Operational Safety, Health and Welfare) Regulations 1976 [43][1]

These Regulations make general provisions for ensuring the safety and health of persons on offshore installations by requiring, inter alia, the control of dangerous substances [44], the maintaining and testing of equipment [45], the independent examination of lifting gear [46], the guarding of dangerous machinery and apparatus [47], and require that 'at all times all reasonably practical steps shall be taken to ensure the safety of persons [48].' In particular, any area in which there is a likely danger of fire must be marked as a 'hazardous area' and shown on drawings comprised in the operations manual for an offshore installation [49]. Further, no work giving rise to a source of ignition (such as welding), or on electrical equipment, or giving rise to noxious gases where there is inadequate ventilation, may be conducted save by a competent person and in accordance with the instructions of the installation manager [50]. In Schedule 4 to the Regulations, detailed provisions relating to drilling and production operations are set out.

As regards health, an adequate and accessible supply of drinking water must be provided and maintained, and all provisions must be 'fit for human consumption, palatable and of good quality [51]'. On every offshore installation a 'sick bay' must be provided, in an accessible location, and maintained in a good and clean condition [52]. It must be suitable for medical treatment and the care of sick and injured persons, and in its immediate vicinity must be a bath, supplied with adequate hot and cold water, and a water closet [52]. Schedule 5 to the Regulations lists the equipment and the medicines which must be provided and properly stored and marked [52], and one 'medically trained person', or two if there are more than 40 persons on the installation, must be provided [53]. A 'medically trained person' means either a State

---

1. It is anticipated that the relevant parts of these regulations will be incorporated into and replaced by the Offshore Installations and Pipeline Works (First Aid) Regulations 1986 which, after many delays, are due to come into effect at about the time the book is going to press. Their general effect will be to extend and tighten the 1976 regulations. — Editor

Registered Nurse, or the holder of a certificate of competency issued by the St. John Ambulance Association of the Order of St. John, the St. Andrew's Ambulance Association or the British Red Cross Society, provided such persons have received adequate training in the use of mechanical artificial respiration equipment [53].

As already mentioned, it is the duty of the installation manager, the installation owner, and in certain instances, the licensed concession owner, to ensure the regulations are complied with. But it is also the duty of each person on an installation to do nothing to endanger life; to cooperate with his employer; to report any defect in equipment; and to report any dangerous work not being carried out in accordance with written instructions [54]. Any person in breach of a duty imposed by the regulations shall incur civil liability if any personal injury results [55]. Regulation 34 also makes contravention of any of the regulations an offence, unless the offender can show he exercised all due diligence to prevent the offence or that it 'was committed without his consent, connivance or wilful default [56].'

A draft Health and Safety (Offshore Installations and Pipeline Works) First-Aid Regulations, Approved Code of Practice and Guidance Notes [57] have been proposed and are expected to come into force in the last quarter of 1986. The format of draft regulations, supported by a draft approved code of practice and guidance notes, is similar to the Health and Safety (First-Aid) Regulations 1981 [58] which apply onshore. The draft Regulations impose a general duty on the person in control of an offshore installation or barge to make adequate and appropriate first-aid provision for those at work (defined as all workers on the offshore installation whether on or off duty), and to inform all workers of the first-aid arrangements that have been made. The draft First-Aid Regulations would revoke the requirements on first aid on offshore installations contained in Regulations 27 and 31 and Schedule 5 of the 1976 Operational Safety, Health and Welfare Regulations.

The Offshore Installations (Emergency Procedure) Regulations 1976 [59]

These Regulations require the provision of an 'emergency procedure manual' specifying the action to be taken if an emergency, which by definition includes an apprehended emergency, occurs [60]. 'A death, a serious injury or illness' [60] are included as examples of an emergency, as well as fires, blowouts, collisions and similar events [61]. The manual must specify, inter alia, instructions for evacuating the installation, detail the emergency services arranged for divers diving near the installation and detail available search and rescue services and any action arranged by the owner of the installation to be taken by persons onshore or on another installation [62]. The Secretary of State may request a copy of the manual, and order amendments if he considers any provision insufficient [63].

There is also provision for 'musters' [64] and 'practice drills' [65] every 12 days, and the stationing of a safety vessel, capable of safely accommodating and providing first-aid treatment for all persons on the installation, within 5 nautical miles of the installation [66]. Apart from the installation owner, the licensee concession owner and the installation manager all having a duty to ensure the regulations are complied with, every person on the installation also has a duty 'to acquaint himself with his emergency station and any duties assigned to him in the event of an emergency [67].' The position with regard to failure of a person to discharge his statutory duty is as mentioned in the Operational Safety, Health and Welfare Regulations.

The Offshore Installations (Inspectors and Casualties) Regulations 1973 [68]

These Regulations empower an inspector to board and gain access to an offshore installation at any time, and there to test or examine any equipment and require any person to act or not to act [69] in order to avoid or minimise a 'casualty', defined as a 'casualty or other accident involving loss of life or danger to life' to a person on the installation or an attendant vessel [70]. The purpose of the power is not just to permit investigation of an accident, but also to ensure the provisions of the 1971 Act are being complied with, and the ancillary powers given to an inspector to require production of documents or information are wide [71].

The regulations also deal with the monitoring of all 'casualties' [70]. The manager must immediately notify the owner of the installation following a casualty, detailing the time it occurred and the identity of the person killed, lost, or seriously injured, and within 3 days thereafter deliver further particulars [72]. The owner must also inform the Secretary of State for Industry of the casualty and provide him with a copy of the further particulars furnished by the installation manager [73], and the site of any casualty must not be disturbed until 3 days after the Secretary of State is notified, unless an inspector has attended earlier [74]. In addition, the owner must make a quarterly return [75] to the Secretary of State for Industry of every other accident, injury or disease which caused a person to be unable to work for a period of 3 consecutive days [76]. Breach by the manager or owner of the above-mentioned duty is an offence under the 1971 Act.

In relation to any casualty or other accident involving loss of or danger to life, the Offshore Installations (Public Inquiries) Regulations 1974 [76] allows the Secretary of State to hold a public inquiry, and the person appointed to hold the enquiry has wide powers to enable him to conduct the inquiry [77].

The Diving Operations at Work Regulations 1981 [78]

These are the principal Regulations applicable to any diving operations, though any diving operations in connection with pipeline works on the continental shelf are also covered by the Submarine Pipelines (Diving Operations) Regulations 1976 [79].

It is the duty of the diving contractor or any person who has control over the divers, and the duty of the owners of any offshore installation or pipeline to ensure, so far as is practicable, that the Regulations [80] are complied with and not to expose persons in any way to risks to their health and safety. Every diving contractor, in respect of each diving operation, must: appoint one or more qualified diving supervisors; keep an operations logbook; ensure operations are carried out from a suitable and safe place; and that emergency services and facilities for transferring persons for treatment are available (including saturation techniques) [81]. All divers must have a valid certificate of training and medical fitness [82], the latter to be issued by an approved doctor or by the Health and Safety Executive [83], and a personal logbook in which a daily record of diving is recorded [82]. The certificate of medical fitness shall specify a period, not to exceed 12 months, for which the diver is considered fit and the certificate is entered into the diver's personal log.

Whenever a diving operation is to be carried out there must be a diving team present, including a stand-by diver, able to ensure that the operation is carried out safely and able to operate all equipment and machinery [84]. The diving contractor must formulate diving rules [85] to be given to the diving supervisor and be available on demand to any inspector [86]. The Regulations also provide for certain plant and equipment to be available, and properly tested and maintained [87]. It should also be mentioned that comprehensive guidance notes have been issued by the health and safety executive in relation to diving operations covered by the regulations.

The Petroleum and Submarine Pipelines Act 1975

Under the Petroleum and Submarine Pipelines Act 1975 [88] the Secretary of State may, by regulations, provide for the safe operation of pipelines and the safety, health and welfare of persons engaged on pipeline works. The 1975 Act contains provisions very similar to the Mineral Workings (Offshore Installations) Act 1971 discussed above, in that regulations may provide for the holding of public inquiries into accidents connected with pipelines, and inspectors, appointed by the Secretary of State in relation to such public inquiries, may be granted powers of entry, of summoning witnesses and of ordering the production of documents [89]. To avoid any conflict between the regulations issued under the Mineral Workings (Offshore Installations) Act 1971 and the 1975 Act, pipelines forming part of an offshore installation [90] are excluded from the 1975 Act [91]. At present the only regulations issued pursuant to Section 26 of the 1975 Act are Submarine Pipelines (Diving Operations) Regulations 1976, the contents of which complement the Diving Operations at Work Regulations 1981, discussed above, and the Submarine Pipelines Safety Regulations 1982 [92].

The Health and Safety at Work etc. Act 1974 ('the 1974 Act')

The provisions of Parts I, II and IV of the Health and Safety at Work Act 1974 apply to certain activities on the United Kingdom continental shelf by virtue of the Health and Safety at Work etc. Act 1974 (Application outside Great Britain) Order 1977 [93], and that Order also extends to territorial waters the provisions of the 1974 Act relating to construction and diving operations.

The 1977 Order applies to offshore installations [94] and to activities carried out on and from an offshore installation, or from a vessel in relation to such an installation, but does not apply to aircraft [95]. The activities covered include diving operations [96], and the activities of any person connected therewith; inspection; testing; loading and unloading; fuelling; provisioning; construction; repair work; maintenance; cleaning; demolition; and all operations in relation to the survey and preparation of the seabed for an offshore installation [97]. The Order also extends the Act to pipeline works [98] which includes assembling, placing, inspecting, repairing, and removing of a pipeline, as well as diving operations connected with a pipeline and also related activities such as unloading, fuelling, repairing and maintenance of a vessel or aircraft used in connection with such pipeline works. Within territorial waters, the 1974 Act applies to construction and dismantling of any building or vessel; the loading or unloading of any vessel; and diving operations connected with a building or vessel [99].

Any offence under Section 33 Part 1 of the 1974 Act committed on the continental shelf is treated as an offence within the United Kingdom [100]. Part I generally covers health, safety and welfare in connection with work and the control of dangerous substances. It places duties on employers to ensure, 'as far as is reasonably practicable', that places of work, and methods used, are safe and without risk to health [101]. Even employees have a statutory duty to take reasonable care, and to cooperate with their employer to enable the latter to comply with his statutory duties [102]. Enforcement of the 1974 Act and regulations thereunder is provided for through the appointment of inspectors [103]. Section 33 makes it an offence to contravene the 1974 Act or any health and safety regulations, and officers of a body corporate may incur personal liability if their consent or connivance to the offence can be established. Part II of the Act provides for the continuance of the Employment Medical Advisory Service [104], which is concerned with advising the Secretary of State, employed persons and others on health in relation to employment and training.

Employer's Liability Insurance Offshore

In 1969 the Employer's Liability (Compulsory Insurance) Act was passed, coming into force on 1 January 1972, which imposed on every employer carrying on business in Great Britain a duty to insure and maintain insurance against liability for bodily injury or disease sustained by employees, and arising out of and in the course of their employment in Great Britain. The insurance policies have to be 'approved' [105] and the insurers 'authorised' [105], both as provided in the 1969 Act, and the amount to be insured is currently set at £2 million in respect of claims of any one or more employees arising out of any one occurrence.

Pursuant to Sections 6 and 7 of the Mineral Workings (Offshore Installations) Act 1971, and paragraph 4(b) of the Schedule thereto, the Offshore Installations (Application of the Employer's Liability (Compulsory Insurance) Act 1969) Regulations 1975 [106] were issued. These Regulations amended the 1969 Act by deleting the limitation to employment in Great Britain, and substituting references to

> relevant employees who are employed . . . for work on or from a relevant installation, or on or from an associated structure in the course of any operation undertaken on or in connection with a relevant installation [107].

A 'relevant installation' means an offshore installation to which the 1971 Act applies and an 'associated structure' means a vessel, aircraft, hovercraft or any floating structure used in connection with the installation. A 'relevant employee' means a person ordinarily resident in the United Kingdom or, if not, a person on a 'relevant installation' or 'associated structure' for a continuous period of 7 days [108].

As with other regulations, the licensee concession owner and the owner of the installation are responsible for ensuring compliance, and it is an offence to fail to do so unless it can be shown that all 'due diligence' to prevent the commission of an offence was exercised and contravention was without the respective owner's consent, connivance or wilful default [109]. Also, a company and its officers may be liable as prescribed in the 1971 Act [110] for breach of these Regulations, and any employer of a 'relevant employee' is liable to a fine if the Regulations are not complied with [111]. Each employer of a 'relevant employee' must ensure that a copy of the relevant certificate of insurance is maintained on the 'relevant installation' or 'associated structure' and must be produced on the reasonable request of any 'relevant employer [112].'

Summary

It can be seen that in a short period of time a wide and comprehensive body of legislation has been built up to govern safety, health and welfare offshore the United Kingdom. Further, the application of legislation to concession owners, offshore installation owners and all working on or from an offshore installation means that all concerned with offshore operations have a potential exposure to liability. Any contravention will, per se, be an offence unless it can be shown that it was committed without a person's consent, connivance or wilful default. This potential liability is a serious concern of offshore operators, who consequently must ensure that contractors engaged on offshore installations comply at all times with the legislative requirements.

It would be remiss in considering the legal aspects of safety, health and welfare to refer only to statutory liability, and not to touch on the problem of tortious liability arising from accidents. As already mentioned [113], the civil laws of England, Scotland and Northern Ireland have been extended to the continental shelf, thereby permitting injured persons to recover damages against any tortfeasor. However, what is of greater concern and more problematical to persons operating offshore is the risk of litigation being commenced in the United States, where litigation is more common and damages awarded are substantially higher than in the United Kingdom.

The oil industry's close association with the United States, through licensee companies, contractors and their respective employees, increases the likelihood of United States litigation arising out of an accident on the United Kingdom continental shelf. In a recent decision a plaintiff was held to be entitled to discontinue proceedings brought in England so as to permit him to file suit in the United States with the prospect of greater damages being awarded [114], a decision which appears to condone forum shopping. Offshore oil workers employed aboard drilling rigs and drill ships, and contributing to the function of the vessels, have been held to be seamen [115] and, as such, entitled to the remedies afforded by the Jones Act and the general maritime laws of the United States. The Jones Act is not limited in its application to United States citizens, but provides a remedy to all seamen injured in the course of their employment [116]. However, the Jones Act has now been amended to exclude foreign aliens engaged in the exploration, development or production of natural resources in the territorial waters or continental shelf of a nation, from bringing an action under the Act or any other maritime law of the United States. The only exception is if the person bringing an action has no remedy in the nation in whose jurisdiction the incident occurred or in the nation of which such person is a citizen or resident [117].

For a claim to be brought in the United States for a tort committed abroad, it must first be determined if United States courts have jurisdiction, and in that regard particularly whether the defendant had sufficient contact with a particular State for it to be fair and reasonable in all the circumstances for that State to assume jurisdiction over the defendant [118]. It has been held by the Supreme Court of the United States that, in determining if United States courts have jurisdiction to hear a claim, regard will be had to, inter alia:

The place of the tort
The law of the vessel's flag
The domicile of the injured person
The allegiance of the defendant shipowner
The place of the injured person's contract of employment or articles
The inaccessibility of the foreign forum
The law of the forum [119]

However, the United States Supreme Court in *Lauritzen* concluded that the law of the flag should govern maritime torts, unless there were strong reasons to hold otherwise, such as, that the flag is one of convenience [120], and the willingness of the courts to look to the reality of the situation is reflected in the decision in *Rhoditis* [121]. Here, the United States Supreme Court accepted jurisdiction in an action brought by a Greek seaman, employed in Greece under Greek articles, injured in New Orleans while aboard a Greek-registered vessel, flying the Greek flag and owned by a Greek corporation. In arriving at its decision, the Court attached considerable importance to the fact that the shipowner's base of operation was in the United States.

Even if it is decided that the United States courts have jurisdiction to hear a claim, it must also be considered whether the courts are the proper forum to hear the claim or whether another forum would be better suited. In a recent case [122] a trial judge refused to hear a claim against a United States aircraft manufacturer on the grounds of *forum non conveniens*, and the United States Supreme Court upheld the exercise by the trial judge of his discretion, notwithstanding that the claimant was prejudiced by the laws of the other jurisdiction and that the damages recoverable would be smaller [123].

It appears that more recently the United States courts have been less willing to assume jurisdiction [124] and to hear claims when an effective remedy is available in another jurisdiction which has more nexus with the incident giving rise to the claim, as, for example, residence of witnesses and claimants. However, the risk of persons connected with offshore installations becoming involved in litigation in the United States courts is a very real one, particularly in respect of incidents involving United States citizens, and clearly any action would be substantially facilitated for the claimant if an offence under applicable United Kingdom regulations has been committed. This problem of exposure to tortious liability in the United States is discussed further in Chap. 4 with regard to medical practitioners practising medicine offshore.

References

1. In 1609, James I issued a proclamation excluding Dutch fishermen from fishing off the shores of England
2. See *R v Kent Justice, ex parte Lye* (1967) 2 Q.B. 153; (1967) 2 W.L.R. 765
3. Full title is 'Convention on the Territorial Sea and The Contiguous Zone. Done at Geneva, on 29 April, 1958'
4. Article 24 (1)
5. Article 24 (2)
6. Full title is 'Convention on the Continental Shelf. Done at Geneva, on 29 April, 1958'
7. Article 2 (1)
8. Article 1. On the high seas each nation, in particular, has freedom of navigation, fishing, laying of pipeline and cables, overflying, but in the exercise of such freedom must take into account the interests of other states — see Article 2 of the Geneva Convention on the High Seas
9. Article 1 of the Convention on the High Seas. Done at Geneva, on 29 April, 1958; defines the high seas as 'all parts of the sea that are not included in the territorial sea or the internal waters of a State'
10. See Article 2 of the Convention on the High Seas
11. Full title is 'Convention on the Continental Shelf. Done at Geneva, on 29 April, 1958'
12. See the 'North Sea Continental Shelf' Case ICJ Rep, 1969 p 1
13. See reference 12
14. Section 1 (1)
15. For definition of petroleum see Section 1 (2) of the Petroleum (Production) Act, 1934
16. Section 1 (3), the rights onshore are granted by Sections 2 and 6 of the Petroleum (Production) Act 1934. Section 2 provides for the granting of licences, and Section 6 for the making of regulations pertaining to such licences

17. Section 1 (4)
18. Section 1 (7)
19. See Continental Shelf (Designation of Areas) Orders: SI 1964 No. 697; SI 1965 No. 1531; SI 1968 No. 891; SI 1971 No. 594; SI 1974 No. 1489; SI 1976 No. 1153; SI 1977 No. 1871; SI 1978 No. 178; SI 1978 No. 1029; SI 1979 No. 1447
20. SI 1968 No. 892, as amended by the Continental Shelf (Jurisdiction) (Amendment) Orders 1980 and 1982; SI 1980 No. 184; SI 1980 No. 559; and SI 1982 No. 1523
21. See Sections 21,22,23,37 and Schedule 4 to the Oil and Gas (Enterprise) Act 1982
22. Note: although discussion is with regard to the 'continental shelf', the Mineral Workings (Offshore Installations) Act 1971 and regulations thereto, discussed below, apply also to territorial waters, see Section 8 of the 1971 Act
23. See reference 16
24. For licences issued after 20 August 1976, the model clauses are contained in Schedule 5 of the Petroleum (Production) Regulations 1976; and for earlier licences, in Schedule 2 to the Petroleum and Submarine Pipelines Act 1975
25. The Secretary of State for Energy
26. Model Clause 24 of the licences referred to in reference 23
27. Model Clause 1 (2) of the licences referred to in reference 23
28. Model Clause 22 of the licences referred to in reference 23
29. The original Section 1 has been submitted by a revised Section 1 set out in Section 24 of the Oil and Gas (Enterprise) Act 1982. See also Section 44 of the Petroleum and Submarine Pipelines Act 1975
30. Section 1 (2) as substituted and revised
31. Section 3 (4)
32. Section 44 (1) and (2) Petroleum and Submarine Pipelines Act 1975
33. Section 4 (1). See Offshore Installations (Managers) Regulations 1972 SI 1972 No. 703
34. Section 5 (1) and (2)
35. Section 5 (6)
36. Section 5 (5)
37. Section II, which provides that reference in Section 1 of the Fatal Accidents Act 1976 as it applies to a wrongful act, neglect or default shall include references to any breach of duty actionable by virtue of the 1971 Act
38. Section 7. An offence may be punished on a summary conviction by a fine not exceeding £400, and on conviction on indictment by a term of imprisonment of up to 2 years, a fine, or both. See discussion of regulations below
39. Section 10 (3)
40. Section 9
41. The Offshore Installation (Registration) Regulations 1972 SI 1972 No. 702; the Offshore Installations (Logbooks and Registration of Death) Regulations 1972, SI 1972 No. 1542; the Offshore Installation (Inspectors and Casualties) Regulations 1973, SI 1973 No. 1842; the Offshore Installations (Construction and Survey) Regulations 1974, SI 1974 No. 289; the Offshore Installations (Public Inquiries) Regulations 1974, SI 1974 No. 338; the Offshore Installations (Application of the Employers' Liability (Compulsory Insurance) Act, 1969) Regulations 1975, SI 1975 No. 1289; the Offshore Installations (Operational Safety, Health and Welfare) Regulations 1976, SI 1976 No. 1019; the Offshore Installation (Emergency Procedures) Regulation 1976 SI 1976 No. 1542; the Offshore Installations (Life-Saving Appliances) Regulations 1977, SI 1977 No. 486, as amended by SI 1978 No. 931; the Offshore Installations (Fire Fighting Equipment) Regulations 1978, SI 1978 No. 611; the Offshore Installations (Well Control) Regulations 1980 SI 1980 No. 1759; the Offshore Installations (Lifesaving Appliances and Fire Fighting Equipment) (Amendment) Regulations 1982 SI 1982 No. 360 (Amending SI 1977 No. 486 and SI 1978 No. 611); the Offshore Installations (Application of Statutory Instruments) Regulations 1984 SI 1984 No. 419
42. Offshore Installations (Application of Statutory Instruments) Regulations 1984, SI 1984 No. 419
43. SI 1976 No. 1019
44. Regulation 4
45. Regulation 5
46. Regulation 6
47. Regulation 12
48. Regulation 14
49. Regulation 2
50. Regulation 3
51. Regulation 26
52. Regulation 27
53. Regulation 31

54. Regulation 32
55. Regulation 33 provides that Section II of the Mineral Workings (Offshore Installations) Act 1971 applies to any duties imposed on persons by the Regulations. See reference 12
56. Regulation 34
57. Health and Safety Commission, Consultative Document, H.M. Stationery Office
58. SI 1981 No. 917
59. SI 1976 No.1542
60. Regulation 4 (1)
61. Regulation 4 (1) (6)
62. See generally, Regulation 4 (2) and (3)
63. Regulation 4 (7)
64. Regulation 7
65. Regulation 8
66. Regulation 10
67. Regulation 11 (c)
68. SI 1973 No.1842
69. See generally, Regulation 2 (1)
70. See definition in Regulation 1
71. See generally Regulations 3 and 4
72. Regulation 9
73. Regulation 10
74. Regulation 11, but see defences in Regulation 14
75. Regulation 12
76. SI 1974 No. 338
77. See generally, Regulations 4, 5, 6 and 7. See also obligation to make a return of any death or person lost in Offshore Installations (Logbooks and Registration of Death) Regulations 1972, SI 1972 No. 1542
78. SI 1981 No. 399
79. SI 1976 No. 923. Essentially overlap with 1981 Regulations (see Section 25 Oil and Gas (Enterprise) Act 1982)
80. Section 4. Includes owners of proposed installations or pipelines
81. Section 5
82. Section 7
83. Section 11
84. Section 8
85. Section 9
86. Under the Health and Safety at Work etc. Act 1974
87. Sections 12 and 13
88. Section 26
89. Section 27
90. As the definition is extended by Section 44 of the Petroleum and Submarine Pipelines Act 1975
91. Section 26 (3)
92. SI 1982 No. 1513
93. SI 1977 No. 1232
94. Section 4. Similarly defined as under the Mineral Workings (Offshore Installations) Act 1971 and excludes installations forming part of a pipeline
95. Section 3
96. Section 2 (3)
97. Section 4
98. Section 5
99. Section 7
100. Section 8 (1). Note: Section 8 (2) provides that Section 3 of the Territorial Waters Jurisdiction Act 1978 does not apply to an offence under the 1974 Act
101. See generally, Sections 2–9, Health and Safety at Work etc. Act 1974
102. Section 7, Health and Safety at Work etc. Act 1974
103. Sections 18–26, Health and Safety at Work etc. Act 1974
104. Established under the Employment Medical Advisory Services Act 1972
105. Section 3 (a) and (b), Employers' Liability (Compulsory Insurance) Act 1969
106. SI 1975 No. 1289
107. Section 3 (a), SI 1975 No. 289
108. Definitions: see generally, Section 1 (2), SI 1975 No. 289
109. Section 6

110. As reference 39
111. Section 6
112. SI 1975 No. 1289
113. SI 1975 No. 1289
114. See *Castanho* v *Brown and Root (UK) Ltd and Another* (1980) 3 W.L.R. 991
115. See *Gianfala* v *Texas Co.* 350 U.S. 879 (1955)
116. See also the United States Death on the High Seas Act 41 Stat 537; 46 U.S.C.A. 761
117. Jones Act, 46 U.S.C. 688, amended effective 29 December 1982
118. The Due Process Clause in the 14th Amendment to the U.S. Constitution
119. *Lauritzen* v *Larsen* 345 U.S. 571 (1953)
120. See *Bartholomew* v *Universe Tankships, Inc* 263 F.2d 437 (2nd Circ. 1959) cert denied 359 U.S. 1000
      (1959)
121. *Hellenic Lines* v *Rhoditis* 398 U.S. 306 (1970)
122. *Piper Aircraft Co* v *Gaynell Reyno* pers. rep. of estate of William Fehilly et al. 8 December 1981, 454
      U.S. 235
123. The other forum was Scotland where there was no strict liability and the claimant had to show
      negligence on the part of the aircraft manufacturer.
124. See reference 124 and *Alexander Kielland Claimants* v *Phillips Petroleum Company Norway* where
      the Northern District Court for Ohio refused to accept jurisdiction in respect of an accident arising
      on Norway's continental shelf, a decision affirmed by the U.S. 6th Circuit Court of Appeals, and the
      U.S. Supreme Court in 1984

Schedule of Principal Legislation Governing Safety, Health and Welfare Offshore in Denmark, France, The Netherlands and Norway

Set out below are references to the principal legislation governing safety, health and welfare offshore in Denmark, France, Netherlands and Norway. The references are not intended to be exhaustive and refer primarily to the enabling laws.

Denmark

1. *Subsoil Act* (Lov om Anvendelse af Danmarks Undergrund) Ministry of Energy, Act No. 293 of 10 June 1981

2. *Act on Certain Marine Installations* (Lov om Visse Havanlaeg) Ministry of Energy, Act No. 292 of 19 June 1981

3. *Act on the Protection of the Marine Environment* (Lov om Beskyttelse af Havmiljoeet) Ministry of Environment, Act No. 130 of April 1987

4. *Statutory Order on the Use of Oil Journals* (Bekendtgoerelse om Anvendelse af Oliejournaler) Ministry of Environment S.O. No. 420 of 7 September 1983

5. *Statutory Order on the Coordination Committee for Offshore Installations* (Bekendtgoerelse af Forretningsorden for Koordinationsudvalget) Ministry of Energy S.O. No. 508 of 28 October 1983

6. *Statutory Order on Reporting in Accordance with the Act on the Protection of the Marine Environment* (Bekendtgoerelse om Indberetning i Henhold Til Lov om Beskyttelse af Havmiljoeet) Ministry of Environment S.O. No. 311 of 12 June 1981

7. *Statutory Order on Discharge into the Sea of Substances and Materials from Certain Marine Installations* (Bekendtgoerelse om Udledning i Havet af Stoffer og Materialer Fra Visse Havanlaeg) Ministry of Environment S.O. No. 394 of 17 July 1984

rance

. Code Minier (Articles 77-A-90) Décret 56–838 du 16 août, 1956 and Loi 77-620 du 16 juin, 1977
. Code du Travail
. Circulaire IG-H.S.M. No. 94 due 27 juillet, 1954: Sécurité des Travaux de Forage pour la recherche et l'exploitation d'hydrocarbures liquides et gazeux
. Décret No. 59-285 due 27 janvier, 1959 (modifié): Règlement Général sur l'exploitation des mines autres que les mines de combustibles, minéraux solides et les mines d'hydrocarbures exploités par sondage
. Décret No. 62-725 due 27 juin, 1962: Règlement de sécurité des travaux de recherche par sondage et d'exploitation par sondage des usines d'hydrocarbures liquides et gazeux
. Loi No. 68-1181 du 31 décembre, 1968 (modifié par loi No. 77-485 due 11 mai, 1977): Exploitation due plateau continental et exploitation des ses ressources naturelles
. Décret No. 72-645 due 4 juillet, 1972: Mesures d'ordre et de police relatives aux recherches et à l'exploitation des mines et carrières
. Décret No. 76-48 due 9 janvier, 1976; Protection due personnel dans les mines et carriers qui mettent en oeuvre des courants électriques

letherlands

Aijnwet Continentaal Plat 1965 (Mining Law Continental Shelf)

rticle 26 of the above law authorises legislation to be issued covering the protection f safety and health of persons employed in mining activities, and the health and afety rules issued pursuant thereto are embodied in *Mijnreglement Continentaal 'lat 1967* (Mining Regulations Continental Shelf) as amended

lorway

. *Regulations of Maritime Directorate issued on 10 September 1973*. Covers mobile Drilling Platforms with installations and equipment used for drilling for petroleum in Norwegian internal waters, Norwegian territorial waters and in that part of the continental shelf which is under Norwegian sovereignty
'. *Royal Decree of 3 October 1975*. Contains regulations relating to safe practices etc. on fixed installations relating to exploration and drilling for submarine petroleum resources
'. *Royal Decree of 9 July 1976*. Contains regulations relating to the production, etc. of submarine petroleum resources from fixed installations
'. *Work Environment Act, 4 February 1977*. Covers safety and protection of employees offshore and onshore and on both fixed and mobile installations, pursuant to which regulations have been issued covering work offshore, including the *Royal Decree of 1 June 1979* covering protection of workers and the control of the working environment of all persons working in connection with submarine

5. *Royal Decree of 25 November 1977*. Relates to hygiene, medical equipment and medicines, etc. on installations for production, etc. of submarine petroleum resources

This was in part amended by the Petroleum Activities Act No.11 of 22 March 1985.

Chapter 3

Pre-placement and Periodic Medical Examinations

R.A.F. Cox

Pre-placement Examinations

The main purpose of any pre-placement medical examination is to ensure that the potential employee is medically suited to the proposed employment. If the employment is at a remote offshore location, this factor must be taken into account, in addition to the medical requirements of the job itself. It is important to detect and exclude potential workers who may have some disease or disability which could endanger their lives in an isolated situation, or could develop into an acute medical emergency requiring urgent evacuation ashore.

As will have been appreciated from Chap. 1, offshore work is not suitable for anyone who is not 100% fit, nor for anyone whose working capacity is restricted — there is no provision for part-time work offshore. Drilling rigs and barges do not carry spare quarters and there is no room for a man who cannot play his full part as a member of the team. It follows therefore that anyone sick or injured who is unable to work for more than about 24 h must come ashore, if only to make room for his replacement. This may be very expensive, both for the individual in terms of his loss of earnings and for the employer in terms of working hours lost, plus the direct cost of the evacuation and the cost of replacing the man, either permanently or temporarily.

Not only can an emergency evacuation be expensive for the company, it may also be dangerous. Evacuating a sick man in bad weather conditions may well endanger the crew of the helicopter and others. Some emergencies will arise which no pre-employment medical examination, however comprehensive, could possibly prevent. However, there are many conditions which can cause emergency situations and which are easily detected in the course of a proper pre-placement medical examination.

Furthermore, there are times when offshore installations may be totally isolated by bad weather, so that a condition which may not be life-threatening if the patient can reach hospital in a matter of hours may well become a matter of dire emergency when it is impossible to move the patient ashore for 48 h or more.

The Health and Safety at Work Act, which applies equally to activities offshore and onshore, imposes upon employers a responsibility to maintain the highest standard of health, safety and welfare of all personnel.

> Part I, paragraph 2 (1): It should be the duty of every employer to ensure so far as is reasonably practicable the health, safety and welfare at work of all his employees.

Part II, paragraph 2 (e): The provision and maintenance of a working environment for his employees that is, so far as is reasonably practicable, safe, without risk to health and adequate as regards facilities and arrangements for their welfare at work.

The company has an even greater responsibility in this respect as far as offshore personnel are concerned: (a) because the company is responsible for them 24 h per day while they are offshore; and (b) because they are working in a location far removed from normal medical facilities.

Furthermore, the oil industry in general, and the offshore industry in particular, bear more than their fair share of much emotive criticism for a variety of reasons. In these circumstances, it is clearly prudent that they should not provide further, and perhaps justified, opportunities for such criticism by failing to take all reasonable precautions over the medical screening of their personnel.

The new Offshore Installations and Pipeline Works (first-Aid) Regulations come into effect in 1986 (Appendix 8). In the Guidance notes to these Regulations it is stated that the special conditions of work offshore require workers to be in sound health. All potential offshore employees, therefore, should be examined and given a certificate of fitness by the examining doctor. This can then be produced, on request, at the point of embarkation. Such a certificate is required by law in Norway.

There are certain categories of employees who may be exposed to specific hazards, such as radiation, noise or drilling mud, or in whom some medical conditions could be a risk to others, such as food handlers and crane drivers. Certain additional criteria of fitness may need to be applied to these groups over and above those required for offshore work alone.

The financial attractions of the offshore industry are such that some potential employees with disqualifying medical conditions go to considerable lengths to conceal their disabilities. The fact that a candidate signs a statement acknowledging that a false declaration will result in his dismissal is no deterrent; the doctor must be on the alert for this. The examiner must ask detailed questions about the employee's past history, paying special attention to industrial accidents, compensation which may have been received, and any occasions on which the applicant may have failed a medical examination of any sort or had a life insurance loaded. Two questions which often reveal valuable clues are: (a) 'Have you been off work for any reason at all in the past 2 years?' and (b) 'Are you now taking any tablets, medicines, pills, potions, lotions or any other drugs?'

Enquiries should be made regarding any military service and the medical status of the applicant on discharge. He should also be asked whether he has ever attended hospital or had any X-rays or special investigations.

The answers to all these questions, which should be in writing and signed by the applicant, may give clues to past or present illnesses which may not be revealed until more detailed questioning is pursued by the examiner. If the examiner has any doubts, he should ask the applicant to sign a form giving him permission to approach the applicant's 'own doctor or other relevant medical authority'. If the applicant has been withholding information, this is usually sufficient to produce a voluntary· confession of the whole truth, and, if not, it enables the true facts to be ascertained through the proper medical channels. While this is being done, incidentally, the applicant's employment should be deferred. It is much easier to reject an employee in the first place than to dismiss him on medical grounds later.

The examiner must not be swayed by persuasive pleas by the potential employee whom he has found medically unsuitable. He should explain to the applicant that, in his opinion, he is not suitable for the proposed employment, but that the final decision in the matter will rest with the management, to whom he will make a report.

The doctor does not have executive responsibility in this matter, and acts only in an advisory capacity to the potential employer. He therefore does not have direct responsibility for rejecting unsuitable applicants and, in any case, his advice may be disregarded by the management if the potential employee is so valuable that the company are prepared to accept the medical risk. In deciding upon the employment of a particular person, the project manager has many other factors to take into account apart from the medical ones.

In cases where there is some kind of medical restriction, the doctor's first responsibility is to tell the employers what type of work the patient can safely perform. In the case of offshore workers the employee will either be fit to work offshore or not; there are no half measures, though, in some cases, discretion may be allowed to permit a brief or temporary offshore visit, depending upon the circumstances. He should then explain how his medical condition will restrict his employment, which will give management sufficient nonconfidential data from which they can decide how and where the applicant can be employed. If no such suitable work is available it is their responsibility to inform the applicant. The latter may certainly request a detailed explanation from the doctor, and this should be given without hesitation in the interests of the patient. In most cases where the employee's life or health could be threatened by offshore employment, he will readily accept the doctor's reasoned explanation.

It is unfortunately true, at present, that pre-placement medicals are not mandatory for all companies, especially subcontractors, and since the total offshore work force tends to be drawn from the same 'labour pool', those companies who do not insist on their employees being medically examined tend to employ those who have been rejected by other companies on medical grounds. Some companies therefore become notorious for having medically unfit personnel on their books. These companies are often small outfits doing maintenance, painting, cleaning, and unfortunately, in some cases, catering. The same criteria of fitness should apply to all persons who go offshore, irrespective of their employers.

The UKOOA Medical Advisory Committee (1986) has drawn up fitness guidelines. All offshore workers should be examined in accordance with these guidelines so that a common standard of medical fitness will apply to all offshore employees.

Very close attention should be given to the catering crew, who will require a rather more extensive examination. All food handlers should be carefully examined for any evidence of superficial sepsis, especially in fingers and ears. Special note should be made of personal cleanliness, and they should have a chest X-ray and stool culture. There seems to be little point in performing blood tests for the detection of past venereal disease, though clinical evidence of current infection should be sought. Their examination should be repeated annually or whenever they return from areas such as the tropics, where enteric and other infections are common. An epidemic of enteric fever or food poisoning, however mild, on a rig or barge can be catastrophic, and the cost of any medical examinations to prevent this is a small price to pay.

The evaluation of mental fitness is notoriously difficult and unreliable. Psychometric testing is not accurate enough to determine a man's mental fitness for offshore work, nor will it be practicable to subject each potential offshore employee to such a procedure. Nevertheless, mental equilibrium is of great importance in offshore workers who are subjected to a number of potential causes of stress, e.g.:

1. Regular helicopter flying
2. Family separation

3. Dangers of the work, e.g. potential blowouts, fires
4. Inclement weather
5. The stresses of a small, closed community and, in some cases, tedious and boring jobs

The importance of mental fitness can be appreciated from the fact that, after the first 5 years of operation in the southern North Sea, the North Sea Medical Centre reviewed the reasons for emergency medical evacuations, and acute mental disturbance was second only to trauma. The examining physician should, therefore, formulate a clinical appraisal of the employee's psychological status.

If an employee has been off work through illness or injury, he will require to be seen and reviewed by the company physician, and may require a full, formal, pre-placement examination before it is possible to reach a decision regarding his fitness to return to offshore work. These cases, in particular, must be assessed by a doctor who is familiar with the employee's work environment. Hospital doctors and general practitioners, who have no knowledge of the offshore industry, cannot be expected to know whether a person is fit to return there.

The format of the forms upon which some companies insist that the results of pre-placement physical examinations are recorded leaves much to be desired. They are confused, badly arranged, and cramped; in some cases many of the sections are irrelevant. They are difficult and tedious for the doctor to complete, and it is small wonder that some doctors lose patience and complete the forms without concern for the accuracy of their entries. A form which invites an accurate statement of the facts from the examining doctor must be clear, concise and and as brief as possible. It must, however, be compiled in such a way that the doctor can indicate in a positive manner the result of each aspect of the examination. The clinical findings must be recorded in a way which indicates that each particular part of the examination has in fact been completed. If a doctor has to indicate and append his signature to the specific features of the examination he is not likely to run the medico-legal risk of not actually examining. On the other hand, a statement, 'I have examined Bill Smith and found him fit for offshore work', is no indication that an adequate examination has been performed as the 'examination' is left entirely to the doctor's discretion and may have consisted, regrettably, of only the sight of the patient in the consulting room door.

In those companies which have a medical department, the ultimate responsibility for assessing pre-placement medical fitness will rest with the company's chief medical officer. He, or one of his deputies, will scrutinise these examination forms personally, in which case he will require that the clinical data are properly recorded in a way which enables him to reach his own independent conclusion. A doctor who may be asked by a company without a medical department to perform pre-placement examinations, or to assess examinations done by someone else, should insist that the results of the examination are entered on a form which meets with his approval. If necessary, he should design his own form; he should not accept one which has been compiled by the company's local personnel department. The doctor must return some written indication of the potential employee's physical fitness to the personnel department, but this must not contain any confidential medical data. The form with the clinical data upon it must remain within professional confidence; it must either stay with the examining doctor or be returned to the company's medical department. Forms designed by personnel departments nearly always invite the disclosure of confidential data, which is ethically unacceptable and must be resisted.

The record of the medical status of an employee when he joins the company is an important document, which may be needed for future reference as long as the person remains in employment with the company and, in some cases, for many years afterwards. The time for which these medical documents should be retained is a matter of some debate. The retention of large numbers of files, many containing only a pre-placement medical record, can create a considerable problem in storage space. However, if only for the doctor's own protection, these records should not be destroyed. A reasonable compromise is to store the records of former employees in separate storage boxes, where they are accessible if really necessary, but where they do not take up current filing space. This, however, requires close cooperation with the personnel department and is almost always impossible if the doctor is working for a number of different companies. Microfilming may be the best alternative.

The examination itself will consist of a thorough personal, family, and occupational history, followed by a careful physical examination with the patient adequately undressed. Nowhere is the aphorism 'More mistakes are made by not looking than by not knowing' more true. The urine must be examined for sugar and albumin.

Ancillary investigations are for the most part unnecessary as a routine, but chest X-rays are advisable. They are certainly required for catering personnel and immigrant workers. There is no need for routine blood tests to determine a person's fitness for offshore work, but they may sometimes be clinically indicated before a conclusion can be reached. Catering crews and food handlers should have stool cultures. Where hearing is evaluated a formal audiometry should be done. Any other method of assessing hearing or hearing loss is not accurate or reliable enough to have medico-legal validity.

Apart from caterers and divers (See Chaps. 7 and 8), another group which requires special attention are crane operators, whose binocular vision must be perfect and who must have unrestricted and perfect control over all digits.

The medical standards will vary according to the proposed employment, but a potential employee must not have any condition which could become a hazard to himself or others in the offshore situation.

The following list of possible reasons for not accepting an employee for offshore work is not meant to be comprehensive or totally exclusive, but it hopefully contains all the common conditions likely to be encountered.

1. *Active Peptic Ulceration*. This is an absolute bar from working offshore. If the patient has had adequate medical treatment, healing has been demonstrated by radiology or endoscopy and he has had no symptoms for at least 1 year, or if he has had surgical treatment such as vagotomy and pyloroplasty for the condition, then he may be accepted.
2. *Acute Disease*. Any acute disease, such as current infections, boils, abscesses, and the like, must be corrected before the patient is accepted.
3. *AIDS*. This is definitely unacceptable, but the situation regarding persons who have been discovered incidentally to be carrying the HTLV III virus is less clear. At the present time it is probably reasonable to allow HTLV III carriers to work offshore except as caterers.
4. *Anaemia*. This is a contraindication until its cause has been determined and the condition corrected.
5. *Asthma*. Any person who suffers from recurrent asthma and has had an attack

within the previous 2 years should not be allowed to work offshore. Asthma requiring constant medication for control is not acceptable.

6. *Bronchiectasis*. If purulent sputum is regularly expectorated, bronchiectasis is a bar to offshore work.

7. *Cerebrovascular Disorders*. Any cerebrovascular accident, or a history of a transient ischaemic attack or evidence of general cerebral arteriosclerosis is unacceptable.

8. *Chronic Alcoholism*. Although rigs and barges are supposedly 'dry', chronic alcoholics should not be employed.

9. *Chronic Back Trouble*. Any lesion which causes the patient to have regular time off work is a bar to offshore work. Any patient with a history of back trouble which has necessitated time off work in the previous year should be regarded with considerable suspicion. In all cases of chronic back disease, an X-ray of the lumbar spine should be taken before the patient is accepted.

10. *Chronic Bronchitis*. This condition, when it produces dyspnoea on slight exercise or when the patient regularly has two or more attacks annually for which he needs time off, should disbar a person from offshore work. On standard spirometry the FVC should exceed 70% and the FEV 65% of their predicted values.

11. *Chronic Renal Disease*. This is a bar to offshore work if there is elevation of the blood urea. Urinary obstruction, e.g. from prostatic hypertrophy or urinary incontinence, is a reason for barring offshore employment. Proteinuria must be fully investigated and shown to be orthostatic before acceptance.

12. *Contagious Disease*. Any contagious disease is clearly unacceptable in such a small, closed community as an offshore rig. Perhaps the commonest contagious disease likely to be encountered in these workers is scabies.

13. *Deafness*. A functional hearing loss sufficient to impede normal communication or safety (e.g. inability to hear warning devices) is unacceptable. An intrinsically safe hearing aid may be worn, but the employee must not be dependent on it to hear a safety warning.

14. *Dental Caries*. All dental caries should be corrected before the patient is allowed offshore.

15. *Diabetes*. Insulin-dependent diabetes is an absolute contraindication to offshore work. Some people with maturity-onset mild diabetes, controlled only by diet or minimal oral hypoglycaemic agents, may be acceptable.

16. *Disseminated Sclerosis and Other Neuromuscular or Musculoskeletal Diseases, e.g. Rheumatoid Arthritis*. These are definite contraindications to offshore work.

17. *Drug Addiction*. This is definitely unacceptable.

18. *Ear, Nose and Throat Diseases*. Tympanic membranes should be intact and healthy, though dry perforations may be acceptable. Chronic otitis media or externa is a contraindication for catering crew, and may be a bar to any offshore work if severe. Significant chronic nasal airway obstruction, chronically infected sinuses or frequently recurring sinusitis are generally unacceptable. Recurrent vertigo (Meniere's disease) is a contraindication. Recurrent spontaneous epistaxes should be treated before acceptance. Speech defects may be a bar if they are sufficient to impair safety and efficiency.

19. *Endocrine Disorders*. Endocrine disorders such as acromegaly, thyrotoxicosis, Cushing's syndrome or diabetes insipidus are unlikely to be acceptable for offshore work, unless very stable and well controlled.

20. *Epilepsy*. This is an absolute contraindication to any form of offshore work.

21. *Gallstones*. Except in the case of large solitary stones they are certainly a bar to offshore work.

22. *Gastric Erosion*. Demonstrable healing by endoscopic examination is required before offshore work can be permitted.

23. *Gastrointestinal Diseases*. Patients with ulcerative colitis, colostomy or ileostomies are not suitable. Neither are patients who require special diets.

24. *Gout*. This is only a bar to offshore employment if it is untreated or if the patient cannot be trusted to take his anti-gout therapy regularly.

25. *Gynecological Disorders*. Conditions such as menorrhagia or disabling dysmenorrhoea and pelvic inflammatory disease are unacceptable.

26. *Haemophilia and Other Bleeding Diatheses*. These are definite bars to offshore work.

27. *Haemorrhoids*. If these bleed or prolapse, they should be corrected before the patient is accepted.

28. *Heart Disease*. This is a bar to offshore employment if it is causing symptoms, whether these are controlled by therapy or not. Previous myocardial infarction will not necessarily exclude the patient. If the patient has made a full recovery, has been without symptoms for at least a year, is not receiving specific treatment and has no ECG changes induced by exercise, he may be acceptable. In all cases a specialised cardiological opinion will be required. Coronary bypass surgery will not automatically render an individual fit for offshore work, but persons who have no symptoms and normal exercise tolerance, with a normal ECG, may be acceptable. A current clinical diagnosis of myocardial infarction, angina pectoris or coronary insufficiency is unacceptable, as is symptomatic cardiomyopathy.

29. *Hernias*. Inguinal and femoral hernias may potentially strangulate at any time and workers with such hernias should not be allowed offshore until they have been adequately surgically repaired. A truss is not acceptable. A hiatus hernia is acceptable unless it causes disabling symptoms.

30. *Hypertension*. As a general rule it is reasonable to say that any hypertension which warrants treatment is a contraindication to offshore work. However, exceptions may be made in persons in whom the hypertension is very well controlled by beta blockers or other drugs which do not produce hypotension, and in whom there are no other complications.

31. *Leukemias*. These and other disorders of the reticuloendothelial system, unless in long-term remission, are a contraindication to offshore work.

32. *Liver Disease*. Any liver disease which is sufficient to cause signs or symptoms is a contraindication to offshore work.

33. *Malignant Disease*. Any overt malignant disease is clearly a contraindication, but a person who has had adequate treatment, surgical or otherwise, for a malignant condition and has been totally free of all symptoms or signs of recurrence for 1 year may be considered.

34. *Migraine*. Severe or frequent attacks of disabling migraine will be a cause for rejection.

35. *Musculoskeletal Disease.* There must be no deformity, disability, amputation or prosthesis likely to interfere with normal duties or evacuation procedures.

36. *Nervous Disease.* Any organic nervous disease likely to cause a defect of muscular power, balance, mobility, vision, sensation or coordination is unacceptable.

37. *Obesity.* Anyone who is so obese that his mobility or safety is impaired, bearing in mind that a certain agility is required to transfer from workboats or tugs to barges or climb about the superstructure of drilling rigs, should not be allowed to work offshore until his weight has been adequately reduced.

38. *Pacemakers.* The numerous electric and electronic apparatus offshore may disturb the normal function of pacemakers. Wearers of such instruments should, therefore not usually be permitted offshore, unless they are fitted with fixed rate pacemakers which are now unusual.

39. *Pancreatitis.* Chronic or recurrent pancreatitis is unacceptable.

40. *Pediculosis Corporis and Pediculosis Pubis.* These must be eradicated before a person is allowed offshore.

41. *Peripheral Vascular Disease.* Overt peripheral vascular disease is a definite contraindication.

42. *Pneumothorax.* A history of spontaneous pneumothorax, except for a single episode without recurrence for 1 year, is unacceptable.

43. *Pregnancy.* This is a contraindication to offshore work.

44. *Previous Trauma or Congenital Deformities.* These must be judged on their individual merits and limitations of function according to the employee's job requirement. However, it must be remembered that in any offshore work the employee needs to be agile and mobile.

45. *Psychoses and Many Cases of Neurosis.* These are indications for barring a man from working offshore. If he is sufficiently mentally disturbed that he requires permanent therapy with tranquilisers, antidepressants, or other psychotropic drugs, he should not be accepted for offshore work.

46. *Pulmonary Tuberculosis.* This is unacceptable until treatment is concluded and the attending physician has certified that the patient is no longer infectious.

47. *Regular Drug Therapy.* Those receiving drugs which require careful control or have potentially serious effects, such as anticonvulsants, hypotensives, anti-coagulants, cytotoxic agents, hypoglycaemics, or steroids, are not likely to be acceptable.

48. *Renal Calculus.* This is a relatively common condition, and because of the possible onset of renal colic while a calculus remains in the genitourinary tract, these patients should not be accepted until the calculus has passed spontaneously or been surgically removed.

49. *Renal Disease.* Conditions such as nephritis, nephrosis, polycystic disease, hydronephrosis, renal transplant or nephrectomy with disease in the remaining kidney are unacceptable.

50. *Skin Disease.* Chronic skin disease which may be aggravated by exposure to ultraviolet light, seawater, excessive heat or cold, oil, detergents or other chemicals should be a cause for rejection. So should conditions such as extensive psoriasis, which can be a considerable embarrassment to others in shared sleeping quarters or showers.

51. *Varicocele*. This should be corrected if large enough to cause embarrassment.
52. *Varicose Veins*. These are only a bar where skin changes have occurred and ulceration is overt or imminent.
53. *Venereal Disease*. This also must be treated and cleared before the person is allowed offshore.
54. *Vision*. Correct binocular vision of at least 6/12 is essential for all deck employees. Monocular vision may be acceptable for those engaged in indoor work, such as stewards or radio operators. Chronic glaucoma, uveitis, retinitis pigmentosa, retinal detachment or serious field defects are reasons for rejection. Where spectacles or contact lenses are usually worn, a spare pair must be kept at all times. Proper colour vision is necessary for some categories, e.g. electricians and some operators. Where a colour defect is revealed on testing with Ishihara plates, the prospective employee should be given a vocational colour vision test before acceptance.

Periodic Examinations

In the United Kingdom at the present time, these are voluntary examinations performed as a part of a company's health programme and part of the employment benefits package although the guidelines of the new Offshore Installations and Pipeline Works (First-Aid) Regulations state that it is common practice to ensure fitness through continuing health surveillance. Some companies already make it a mandatory condition for employment for offshore workers at annual or sometimes longer intervals, and in some countries, e.g. Norway, such examinations are obligatory by law on an annual basis. The UKOOA Medical Advisory Committee (1986) guidelines recommend examinations at the following intervals:

Under 40 years of age   3-yearly
42–50 years of age   2-yearly
Over 50 years of age   Annually

The periodic examination is essentially a preventative medical procedure designed to detect incipient disease at an early or pre-symptomatic stage, but it also affords the best opportunity we have at the present time of promoting health education. Periodic examinations are also necessary for any workers who have to meet certain medical standards and included among these, of course, are offshore workers whose medical state is likely to change over the years, and who may well develop conditions which exclude them from such work as they get older.
Special categories include:

1. Food handlers, who should be examined annually and whose examinations should include a chest X-ray and stool culture
2. Crane drivers, in whom particular attention must be paid to binocular vision; They should also be examined annually
3. Employees who work in noisy areas, who should have an annual audiometric examination
4. Workers exposed to ionising radiation, who should be examined annually, but also have a white and red blood count 6-monthly

Because the purpose of a periodic examination is different from that of a pre-placement examination, the content is also rather different. It should include, for example, a review of the employee's work situation and its effects or non-effects upon his health. It is important to ascertain whether he is happy in his work, how much he travels, whether he feels under stress (enquiry must also be made about stress occurring outside work, such as at home) and whether his work involves any unusual or dangerous activities. Personal and family histories are also required to be more detailed. The examination itself will be supported by ancillary tests such as profiles of haematology and biochemistry, chest X-rays, and electrocardiographs in employees over the age of 40.

Most United Kingdom offshore operators now insist on routine periodic examinations, both on their own employees and those of their contractors, and such examinations are legally required in Norway. There must be a fair and equitable system of compensation for those who may be found unfit to continue to work offshore. If the examinations are voluntary, some people who are aware that they have disqualifying conditions do not take the examination, while others who do so and are found unfit are penalised.

As with the pre-placement examination, the medical details are confidential. The company are entitled to know that the person has a condition which may be affecting his work, and in what way, but they are not entitled to know the diagnosis, or any other clinical details. In some cases the examination may reveal a condition or a problem which does not affect the person's current employment, but may have an influence on his future career, e.g. if he were to be given more responsibility, transferred abroad, or moved to some totally different kind of employment within the company. In these cases, the personnel department can be informed that his personal file should be endorsed 'Not to be promoted or transferred without reference to medical'. In this way, management can discuss with the medical department the career changes which they propose before any firm decisions are taken, without the disclosure of confidential medical details.

The patient's general practitioner must be informed of any significant abnormalities which are detected, and of any conditions which may require further follow-up or investigation.

Bibliography

H.M. Stationery Office (1976). The offshore installations and pipeline works (first-aid) regulations, code of practice and guidance notes
Sowton E (1982) Environmental hazards for pacemaker patients. J R Coll Physicians Lond 16 : 159–164
UKOOA (1980) Recommended general medical standards of fitness for designated offshore employees
UKOOA (1985) Environmental health guidelines for offshore installations
UKOOA Medical Advisory Committee (1986) Medical aspects of fitness for offshore work: a guide for examining physicians

Chapter 4

Provision of Back-up Services

R.A.F. Cox and J.N. Norman

The offshore medics must have qualified medical assistance to call upon, for both practical and medico-legal reasons. Such assistance is best provided by local GPs, who need to be energetic, fit and enthusiastic.

General practitioners have the advantage of being generalists who are experienced in dealing with all the most common conditions likely to be encountered. They can easily acquire the additional training, experience and familiarisation with the offshore environment which they will need in due course. General practitioners also have the advantage of being ubiquitous and readily available, without the fixed commitments of surgeons, for example, who cannot always leave their work to attend an emergency. In the normal course of their duties they also provide round the clock cover for their practices, and the additional availability needed for the offshore industry does not require them to compile new rotas or deputising systems. Furthermore, many of the pre-placement routine medical examinations of the offshore employees are likely to have been done by the local GPs, who will thereby have established some rapport with their offshore patients.

Hospital doctors may be required to provide specialist support in some situations. By the very nature of their work, whatever their speciality, they are less readily available than GPs and more constrained by bureaucratic red tape, which makes it more difficult for them to become involved in outside activities, especially those which have such a random demand as offshore emergency medical care. Junior hospital doctors, to whom such duties would normally be expected to fall, have the additional disadvantage of being only temporary in their appointments, which leads to further administrative complications and additional training requirements.

If one or more groups of local GPs are willing to provide the back-up, onshore support, they will need to organise themselves so that one person is available at all times to go offshore for an emergency call. Such a call may take him away from the practice for some hours, so that a 'second on call' system is required to take over practice responsibilities during his absence. Normally it is an advantage if one doctor assumes responsibility for organising the 'on call' rota and ensures that all relevant persons, including the operating companies, helicopter flight controllers, local hospitals, police and other relevant bodies, are informed.

Some form of call-out system is required, and two-way pocket radios are the most convenient. These can either be hand-held or installed in the doctor's car, but the facility of two-way conversation with the base station, where emergency requests are received, is such an asset that the additional cost over other systems such as 'bleeps' is amply repaid (see Chap. 5). However, some of the modern radio-paging devices with facilities for receiving complex messages are now almost as good.

For the great majority of emergencies only one properly equipped doctor will be needed. Rarely, however, in a multiple incident or in a major disaster (see p. 57), additional doctors could be needed and so third, fourth and even fifth reserve doctors may be on stand-by at a lesser stage of readiness. In practice, this usually means either that all members of the emergency team carry their radios and keep them tuned in, or else the first on call must always know the telephone numbers at which his colleagues may be found.

Very rarely a specialist team such as a surgeon with or without an anaesthetist or a mobile intensive care team may be required. Such specialist support should come from the local district general hospital, and it is necessary that the duty doctor should know how to contact and activate such specialist teams.

Any doctor or medical team will need to be properly insured against loss of life or limb. Such insurance can either be provided by the operating company or taken out separately through any aviation insurance brokers. In either case, the terms and conditions of the cover should be agreed and confirmed in writing before an emergency arises and, preferably, included as part of the written contract between the operator and the emergency doctors.

Doctors providing emergency medical support must also ascertain what protection they are receiving for possible indemnity against professional negligence. It must be borne in mind that they themselves may be working on, or giving advice to medics working on, vessels or installations which are outside territorial waters, probably of foreign registration, and containing workers of many nationalities, including American. Furthermore, many of the operating companies will be American owned. In these circumstances some professional indemnity groups decline to cover their members, and separate policies taken out on the open insurance market are prohibitively expensive. In most cases, the operating company will undertake to indemnify the doctor by carrying the risk itself, but it is the doctor's responsibility to ensure that he is protected and, if appropriate, he should insist that he receives a written undertaking to that effect from the operating company. The whole subject has been much influenced by the exorbitant settlements meted out in the American courts, and no doctor should assume that he is automatically protected in these circumstances by his usual professional indemnity policy.

The frequency of emergency calls to the onshore doctors will vary considerably. It will be highest during the initial exploratory phase of an operation, especially if the rigs have new or inexperienced crews, and again during the construction of pipelines and production facilities. There is less fluctuation in the frequency of advice sought by the medics over the radio. Such advice may be required at any time, and the duty doctor must always be readily available to speak to the offshore installation as described in Chap. 5.

It must not be forgotten that the advice tendered to the medic has medico-legal validity, and careful notes of all such conversations should always be kept. Where possible all instructions should be confirmed by telex.

The emergency medical teams may need some refresher training or re-training in techniques of resuscitation, and in some of the specific problems which they may encounter in the offshore situation (see Chap. 6). More importantly, however, they must be familiarised with the offshore environment. This means that each member must visit the offshore installations, whether they be drilling rigs, pipelaying barges or production platforms; they must understand the logistics of helicopter and supply ship operations, and they must be fully familiar with all the channels of communication which they may need to use. Such familiarisation requires some planning and close cooperation between the company's local management and the doctors, but it is an essential requirement if proper medical care is to be provided.

The local physicians will, from time to time, be asked to decide whether an employee who has been off sick or injured is fit to return to work. They cannot offer such an opinion unless they are familiar with the work and the situation.

Although all offshore installations should be well supplied with medical equipment and drugs (see Chap. 5), the emergency doctor will need to take with him a supply of his own. He will have his own particular preference for drugs and dressings in addition to the basic instruments which he will require.

It is better to err on the extravagant side in the selection of equipment, as it is impossible to return for something which has been forgotten, and in almost any emergency visit, the doctor is asked to deal with other problems in addition to the one for which he has been called out.

The equipment should be kept in a special container which may need to be individually constructed for economy of stowage space. This box of equipment should be kept readily available to be put aboard the helicopter when a call for a doctor is received. It is most conveniently kept at the heliport, where it can be put on the aircraft by the ground crew while the doctor is on his way. The box can be kept locked with a combination lock of which the doctors know the number, to avoid the problem created by keys being mislaid.

If the duty doctors' offices are some distance from the heliport or, perhaps, separated from it by a congested town, they may encounter considerable delays and difficulties in getting to the helicopter in an emergency. In these circumstances arrangements should be made for the doctors to be picked up from a selected 'emergency landing site' conveniently close to the doctors' offices. Such arrangements need to be confirmed in advance between the helicopter operators, doctors, local authorities, land owners, police and other affected persons. Similarly, helicopter landing facilities at the local hospital need to be surveyed before they are required in an emergency.

Another necessary training activity for the emergency doctors is that of winching from helicopters. Inevitably, there will be times when a doctor is required on a supply vessel or some structure where there are no helicopter landing facilities. In these circumstances the doctor will have to be winched down, and it is essential that he should be fully familiar with this procedure before he is required to do it in an emergency, and perhaps in inclement weather conditions. Winching up or down from a helicopter looks a rather hazardous procedure but, in fact, it is safe and simple. When it is done over water, the doctor will need to wear an immersion suit and life jacket. The immersion suit must be one of the dry type, and the life jacket of an inflatable pattern which is only blown up if the wearer actually enters the water. The suit must permit unrestricted movement, and should contain sufficient pockets for the doctor to carry his essential instruments without requiring a separate bag or case. It is best if a permanent team is issued with a set of individually fitted and labelled suits specifically for use in all offshore emergencies, including winching. These suits can be kept with the medical gear, and donned either before take-off or while the helicopter is airborne, and before it gets over water. A protective helmet ('bone dome') is also required. Winching, including the winching of stretchers, should be practised regularly, perhaps once or twice per year.

In the organisation of all these activities the respective company medical department should be the instigator. Normally, one of the doctors from the operating oil company's medical department will visit the local doctors and hospitals before his company begins its operations. He will organise the medical support arrangements, ensure that the local medical services, including the hospitals, are aware of the medical implications of the drilling activities, and generally establish the good relations which are necessary between his company, the local contractors and the local medical community, which is certainly going to be greatly affected by any offshore drilling operation. Nothing is likely to sour relationships quicker than a call for help to the local hospital, which may impose a considerable strain on its resources, when no one has even had the courtesy to forewarn them. The establishment of an amicable working relationship between the operating company and the local medical fraternity will go a long way towards establishing friendly relationships with the community as a whole. Once the systems have been established, the day-to-day operations are left to local management and the doctors concerned, with only the occasional visit from a 'head office doctor'.

Some of the members of the emergency medical team may be required to deal with diving problems from time to time. This is a specialised area, dealt with elsewhere in this book (see Chap. 7), but it should be emphasised at this time that such designated members will need special training in hyperbaric medicine. The fact that a doctor may be approved under the Special Diving Regulations to examine divers for their medical fitness does not necessarily mean that he is competent to handle diving emergencies. Before he can be regarded as such, the doctor must have attended at least one approved course in diving medicine. He should also have worked under supervision with a commercial diving organisation or an experimental diving unit and thereby acquired considerable experience in the handling of practical problems of decompression sickness, before he accepts sole responsibility for the management of such cases. Such experience is not easy to come by and requires the expenditure of much time and effort, but it does provide much interesting and convivial activity.

Specialist Services

The organisation of general emergency back-up services has already been described, and such medical organisation takes care of most of the problems which arise. Nonetheless, there is occasionally a requirement for the provision of specialist services for a major offshore disaster. There may also be a need for specialists to attend offshore, either due to the inaccessibility of the patient, as in saturation diving, or because some extrication manoeuvre is necessary. The modern tendency to build large ships to cater for such a disaster as a blowout or fire offshore implies also a requirement for medical specialists to be available to proceed offshore, to care for the injured in the well-equipped facilities with which most of these ships are provided.

In the early 1970s when exploration and construction work was at its height in the northern sector of the North Sea, when the oil companies still had little experience of such work in the remote and hostile conditions of the area and before the emergence of strong safety departments and well-defined training schedules, there were a number of fairly serious traumatic incidents. The potential for a major disaster seemed enormous, and it was felt that it would be difficult to provide adequate medical care for such an event, unless considerable prior preparation and planning had taken place. It seemed clear that a variety of medical specialists had to be recruited and familiarised with conditions offshore, and provided with appropriate equipment kept in a state of readiness for mobilisation. This led to the case being made for the establishment of a series of specialist teams. There have been frequent occasions when specialist advice and help has been required in the management of offshore incidents, but experience has now shown that there is little requirement for an elaborate mobile specialist group. This is partly due to the acquisition of operational know-how by the operating companies and also by the emergence of strong safety and training departments. The personnel have also become much more experienced in work offshore. While this experience was being gained, however, it is a matter of record that there has been no occasion in 10 years in the northern North Sea when the existence of a full specialist team has made any difference to morbidity or mortality, even though there has been a variety of incidents. This is important experience for those who are responsible for providing medical services in new areas of exploration. They will be required to take the same type of decision as those who were responsible for the provision of health and safety in the North Sea during the past decade.

During this time, there has been much thought given to the constitution of the health care team required to cater for the medical problems which arise offshore and also for the provision of such ancillary equipment as may be required. A system has emerged for the provision of medical care for those who work in remote areas, and this includes not only offshore installations, but also such extremely isolated communities as the bases of the British Antarctic Survey. This is based on prior special first-aid training for all those who work in these areas together with the elaboration of special training courses for all members of the health care team. This includes the rig medics and those who are required to escort the seriously ill patients ashore, together with those doctors who require training in specialist areas such as diving medicine and those junior doctors who may work alone for long periods in these isolated situations. This training must be associated with the provision of sophisticated communication devices so that the nurse or the junior doctor offshore acts in many ways as an extension of his specialist colleagues ashore. In this way, it has become possible to manage complex conditions at a distance and to provide the best specialist advice available. At this time new diplomas in remote health care are being promoted, suggesting the added recognition of a new minor specialty.

In the past, areas which supported a substantial degree of offshore workings tended to have groups of doctors who were prepared to provide topside emergency services, a second group for diving emergencies and yet a third group to provide specialist surgical and anaesthetic services. The passage of time and growing experience of providing a high standard of health care for the offshore community suggests that such a system is unnecessarily complex and not very economical. The more recent approach of doctors interested in providing emergency services offshore has been to ensure a variety of skills in their constituent members. All are trained in diving medicine and in addition to general practice, the specialties of surgery, anaesthesia and occupational medicine are represented. This appears to be the most economical and efficient way of providing medical support for offshore emergencies, and the various skills of the constituent members of such a team allow a single efficient service to be provided and to be associated with a very comprehensive system of communications.

Such groups will easily cope with the seriously ill diver in saturation, for example, and also with an offshore disaster which may produce half a dozen seriously ill casualties, but the possible consequences of a major disaster, such as a fire on an offshore installation with many hundreds of casualties, poses a much greater problem. This is a matter of disaster planning which requires the production of a plan for each area similar to major civil disaster plans for onshore situations. Such a plan requires detailed planning and coordination by the responsible authorities which are in a position rapidly to call upon all the resources of the area. In Britain this implies the combined efforts of the Chief Constable of the appropriate city or county together with the Coastguard.

Offshore Disasters

In spite of the most rigorous safety programmes and fail-safe design features, any offshore exploration or production facility is still liable to unforeseen technical problems, human error and environmental hazards, and especially bad weather. For these reasons alone, occasional major catastrophes will occur in the offshore situation as in any other (Fig. 4.1).

The difference between an offshore disaster and an onshore one is mainly logistic. The offshore structure is likely to be isolated, and accessible in an emergency only by helicopter. Assistance of any sort must be transported a considerable distance and may be hampered by the same conditions that may have contributed to the disaster in the first place.

The most likely hazards to produce a major disaster are a blowout (the uncontrolled emission of gas or oil), fire, which may result from a blowout, collision between a ship and a rig, or the foundering or collapse of a rig in a storm. In some operations there may also be a toxic hazard from hydrogen sulphide.

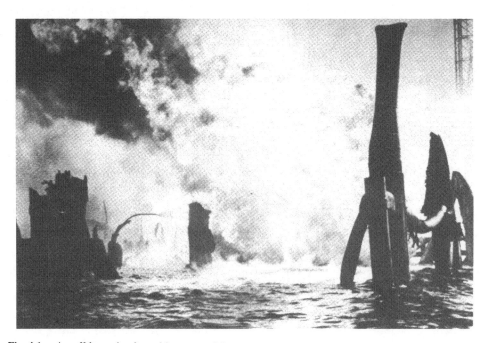

Fig. 4.1.   An offshore rig after a blowout and fire.

In any of these circumstances it is likely that the whole rig or platform will have to be evacuated, and there may be a number of casualties ranging from trivial injuries to death. The total number of people involved may vary from 15 to 25 on the smaller platforms to 300 or more on the large ones and 'flotels'.

As in any other disaster, triage is of paramount importance, but, owing to the limited number of helicopters which will be available, it is impossible to arrange for all the patients to be brought ashore immediately. For this reason it is necessary to establish a medical base on the nearest available and unaffected rig or platform to which a medical team can be taken, and there set up an 'emergency casualty clearing station' where triage can be performed. Every rig or platform must therefore carry sufficient medical equipment to deal not only with any casualties of its own, but with any that it may receive from another rig (see Appendix 4, p. 202).

Effective triage requires adequate space where all the casualties can be sorted. Individual patients in isolated rooms are impossible to keep under proper observation, and are liable to be forgotten. It is therefore essential to keep all the casualties together where the limited number of medical personnel can look after several people at once, and where the less severely injured can lend some assistance while they themselves are kept under observation and documented.

Every rig, therefore, should have one large room (usually the mess or dining room, but it could be a recreation room or even a conference room) which can be rapidly cleared of all its furniture to allow a maximum area of uncluttered floor space for the disposition of stretchers, temporary beds, and even mattresses on the floor for the accommodation of the injured. When new rigs or platforms are designed, such a room should be designated at an early stage so that it can have easy access to the helideck, wide doors, and close proximity to the rig's sick bay (see pp. 67).

In a major disaster situation in which rescue services are organised as described here, triage proceedings can tend to be repeated several times, as exemplified in the Alexander Kielland catastrophe. Here, the casualties were sorted in the hangar on the Ekofisk hotel, again in the conference room, then on arrival at Sola airport in Stavanger, and once more at the local hospital. This repeated sorting could be avoided by the use of record cards, which are attached to or given to each casualty when they are first examined at the first triage point. The card is designed as an *aide-mémoire* so that the essential details can be noted simply by ringing, underlining, or 'ticking' the appropriate titles.

The rig medics will have a critical role to play in any disaster situation, and an early priority of helicopters must be to transport any medics that may be available on nearby rigs to the designated receptor rig. The condition and ultimate survival of any survivors will depend upon the skill of the medic until the arrival of the medical team from ashore.

Cox (1970) has stated:

> In a disaster on land the mobile medical team is taken from the designated hospital. For a disaster at sea, however, it is essential that doctors should be familiar with drilling rigs and their operations and fully conversant with the operation of helicopters and winching. Owing to the constant change of all but senior hospital staff and the fact that drilling operators or shipping agents will have retained the services of local medical personnel anyway, we believe that the members of the emergency medical team should be local general practitioners.

Specialist back-up services provided by the local hospital may well be needed in addition (see p. 54), but the primary mobile medical team is most effectively drawn from the roster of GPs who are providing the daily medical care for the operations. The minimum number of doctors required will be four.

Of the four doctors, one must proceed to the rescue headquarters wherever that has been established. His function is to:

> make all the decisions of a medical nature in connection with the operation, to coordinate the activities of the forward medical teams and to interpret their reports. He will keep the designated hospital informed of the progress of the evacuation, and will notify them when they can 'stand down'. The same medical officer should preferably remain in overall control of the operation until its conclusion (Cox 1970).

His is a vital role. He will establish priorities and will advise the coordinator of the helicopter operations of the urgency and appropriate destinations of casualties. He will act as medical liaison officer between the offshore site and all relevant agencies, including the Press and relatives on shore.

In some disaster situations, two headquarters may be established, one in the operating oil company's office, and the other at the local civilian rescue control centre which may be a heliport, an air traffic control room, a coastguard office, or even a police headquarters. The doctor should be at the company's operations room, where he has access to the maximum amount of incoming information and channels of communication and where he can be of maximum benefit to the other people involved. There should, in any case, be an open line to any other rescue coordinating centre by which the doctor can maintain medical liaison with them. The coordinating doctor onshore must be totally familiar with the offshore operations, and he must therefore be one of the regular doctors. A coordinating doctor drawn, for example, from a local health authority (such as a community physician in England) or the local hospital, will not be sufficiently familiar with the offshore operations to function properly in this role.

At least three doctors should proceed offshore to establish the forward base on the designated receptor rig. Since some casualties may have been picked up by attendant vessels or been transferred to platforms other than the designated receptor platform, the medical team may have to split up, hence the requirement for three doctors. If there are a significant number of casualties then three doctors may well be required on the designated receptor rig alone.

The team of emergency doctors must be familiar with the techniques of being winched from helicopters. They must be trained in this manoeuvre and practise it regularly. The local lifeboat crew usually welcomes the opportunity to participate in these exercises. Frequently, a doctor may have to be winched down to tend survivors on a vessel which may have little or no medical equipment, and the doctor must take his own. The inventory must consist of essential items only, which are stowed in specially constructed boxes fitted with large canvas carrying straps for ease of lowering on the winch wire.

When offshore disaster schemes are planned the local hospitals must be consulted from a very early stage. They will be expected to receive the casualties, and the resources of some local hospitals may be stretched beyond their capacity by a disaster which produces even a moderate number of casualties. In these cases, second or third hospitals may have to be used. Some hospitals are divided, with specialist units such as burns or thoracic surgery at different sites. Helicopter landing facilities may be available at some hospitals, but not all, and arrangements may have to be made with the ambulance service to have enough vehicles available to transfer the casualties.

The role of voluntary organisations in an offshore disaster is very limited. In an onshore disaster, bodies such as the Women's Royal Voluntary Service, the St. John Ambulance Brigade, and the British Red Cross Society can, and do, play most valuable roles. In the offshore situation, however, their potential contribution is very limited, though onshore their help is invaluable in handling the casualties who do not go to hospital or who are quickly discharged. These organisations are always keen to help, and they can provide any number of extra pairs of skilled hands at short notice. Their services can be very valuable in some circumstances; their resources and key personnel should be listed in the disaster plan and their officers should certainly be consulted during its formation.

Though they have an important function in a disaster situation, the Press can be very disruptive to those who are closely engaged with the immediate problems. Normally the public affairs department of the company handles all press enquiries and news releases, but they may be confined to head office and it is necessary to have some appointed representative at the disaster headquarters to deal with the local press relations.

Enquiries from the Press, as well as anxious relatives, can completely swamp the telephone switchboard, so preventing essential calls connected with the rescue operation. In an endeavour to prevent this, a separate enquiry number should be established and broadcast to the public and press as soon as possible. In the United Kingdom responsibility for this function will usually be accepted by the police, who are best equipped to set up such a service and take the pressure off the hospital. This police function should be defined and written into the disaster plan. The police information bureau will be fed by information from police patrol cars at key points, for example helicopter control room, hospital and helicopter landing areas. All possible ex-directory lines should be utilised, and maximum use made of radio communications. An important argument in favour of equipping the emergency doctors with 'walkie-talkie' type radios as opposed to bleeper systems is because of their great value in a disaster situation.

A further aid to communications in a disaster is a private internal telephone line which connects operating oil company offices, helicopter operators' room, police station, hospital and doctor's office. This allows communication between these parties and enables any one of them whose outside lines may be blocked to place a call through one of the others. The line is kept solely for use in such disasters and is not linked directly into the public telephone network.

Any disaster scheme requires regular review and practice. It must be the responsibility of a designated person in the company (usually the safety director or one of his staff) to review the written procedure, checking telephone numbers and names of personnel and correcting them where they have been changed. There may also have been changes in supporting services, such as hospitals, police and fire brigade, which may affect the scheme. The scheme should be reviewed twice a year, the second of these reviews being in fact a paper exercise in which a simulated disaster is worked through in theory. Helicopters, police, hospital services and others involved are contacted as appropriate. Only this type of review will show up gaps and deficiencies, and enable the scheme to be adapted to changing circumstances.

Perhaps every 3 years or so a full-scale simulated emergency exercise should be held to ensure that all the workers involved are fully familiar with their role and functions in a disaster situation.

In such a situation, there may be a small flotilla of vessels acting as rescue ships. Stand-by boats, supply ships, passing coasters and even lifeboats, when the site is fairly close inshore, may all pick up survivors, some of whom may be in urgent need of medical help. It is important that these rescue vessels notify the emergency headquarters of the numbers and names of survivors, so that unnecessary searches are not mounted and so that doctors can be despatched to attend those that need urgent attention.

It is also essential that survivors who appear to be quite uninjured and who may reach another vessel or rig, or even the shore, do not disappear without being medically screened. If they are medically screened, it ensures that they are properly documented and so accounted for, thereby preventing unnecessary searches, but it also ensures that injuries regarded as trivial in the confusion of the disaster do not turn up as more serious ones 24 or 48 h later.

All the survivors brought ashore, however much they protest their fitness, should be taken to the designated hospital for final screening and documentation. Only in this way will an accurate list of survivors (and those missing) be established. An additional reason for taking every survivor to hospital was revealed in the Alexander Kielland disaster. Here much emphasis was placed by Professor Lund (Professor of Catastrophe Psychiatry at the University of Oslo) and his colleagues on the importance of counselling survivors and relatives on the psychiatric disturbances to be expected following a disaster. The psychiatric team are best able to make contact with all the survivors, if only briefly, when they are taken to hospital.

Professor Lund feels that the psychiatric aspects of disasters are neglected, and these factors should be taken into account in the planning for disasters, including offshore ones. He particularly stresses the importance of training doctors and medics who may be involved in the handling of the inevitable psychiatric disturbances which will occur.

Bibliography

British Medical Journal (1975) Medical aspects of North Sea oil. (Editorial) Br Med J III: 576–580

Cox RAF (1970) An Emergency plan for an offshore disaster. Practitioner 205: 663–670

Lancet (1977) Offshore medicine. (Editorial) Lancet II: 751

Levy S, Stoner AG (1977) An offshore medical service at the Cape of Good Hope. S Afr Med J 51: 476–480

Procter DM (1976) Medicine and the North Sea – Hospital support in offshore emergencies. J Soc Occup Med 26: 50–52

Rawlins JS (1977–1978) Medical problems in support of the offshore oil industry. Trans Med Soc Lond 94: 25–32

Scottish Medical Journal (1975) Medical problems of oil development in Shetland. (Editorial) Scott Med J 20: 146–147

Shepherd FGG (1976) Medicine and the North Sea – Emergencies for the general practitioner. J Soc Occup Med 26: 50–52

Chapter 5

Offshore Medical Care

I.K.Anderson and R.A.F.Cox

Functions of the Offshore Medic

In the mid 1960s when oil and gas exploration commenced on the United Kingdom continental shelf, little was known of the medical support needed for this type of operation. While in isolated parts of the world some oil companies had developed sophisticated medical services for their employees working in the field, sparse information appeared to be readily available in the United Kingdom. A large amount of experience had been obtained from military operations in isolated situations where paramedics had been employed, but men with this experience, while valuable, had neither the qualifications nor the right type of experience for a medic in the North Sea. It should also be recalled that in the early days in the North Sea there was little medical screening of offshore workers and some of the medical problems encountered were due to the unsuitability of the work force. Some 20 years' experience in the North Sea has, however, now provided the basis and background for the provision of medical care offshore.

On small gas platforms primary medical care is performed by first aiders, but on larger platforms and other installations such as barges and drilling rigs the work is taken on by medics. While the first aider on small gas platforms is capable of offering considerable assistance in primary care, he is normally only trained in first aid and has some special training in the handling and dispensing of drugs, simple medical record keeping, the transport of patients and problems of immersion. Most of these first aiders in the southern sector of the North Sea are close to medical care and there is no justification for having more experienced people in that position. On a small platform (with 20–30 personnel) it is essential that at least 50% of the men should have received this training and had regular refresher courses. Drilling rigs, barges and oil production platforms should have a certified nurse on board who is a highly trained and designated medic as opposed to the first aiders on the small platforms. (Medics may also be described as sick bay attendants.) Not all drilling rigs have a large number of personnel on board, but the dangerous nature of their work makes it essential that they have a medic. All the medics should hold full nursing qualifications (State Registered Nurse). Qualifications such as State Enrolled Nurse, or those obtained in the armed forces do not appear entirely acceptable on the grounds of experience or from a medico-legal aspect.

A rig medic has the following duties:

1. He (or she) needs to be in attendance on the installation to care for casualties, varying from head injuries, severe trauma and hypothermia to minor cuts and abrasions. This implies that he must know the appropriate primary resuscitative procedures and be capable, for example, of setting up infusions, maintaining an airway or catheterising the bladder.

2. He should start and if necessary continue the treatment of all illnesses offshore. This would include such conditions as upper respiratory tract infections, minor sepsis, skin disorders and dyspepsia. He may have to deal with major medical emergencies, e.g. strokes or myocardial infarction, but it is to be hoped that the medical screening of the offshore population will keep this type of illness down to a minimum. Minor illnesses or accidents not affecting the ability to work should be treated by the medic on site. He will need to know how long somebody can be kept offshore if incapable of work.

3. He has to arrange for the evacuation of injured or sick persons who are not suitable for treatment on board the installation. He must be able to decide on the urgency of the situation and whether a special helicopter medical evacuation is necessary, or whether a routine flight will be suitable. He must be able to decide whether under poor flying conditions it is a justifiable risk to evacuate a casualty. In consultation with a doctor ashore he should be able to decide whether it is necessary for a doctor to fly out to the rig to treat a casualty. It may be necessary when flying is hazardous to treat the casualty offshore under the instruction of the doctor onshore. He must realise the importance of resuscitation and stabilisation prior to evacuation. It is, therefore, important for him to have established a reporting relationship with a group of doctors onshore who are responsible for helping him. He must be aware of the routes of evacuation of casualties and the doctors to be consulted, for both topside and diving medical cover. He must check that his communication system is always efficient.

4. He must be aware of the difficulties and complexities of diving operations and the medical problems associated with diving. He should be prepared to go under pressure and give sensible help to diving supervisors.

5. He must be conversant with his role in a disaster on board the installation and what particular emergency procedure to follow. He must know which hospitals have the necessary facilities to cope with a major disaster and also be aware of the help to be obtained from coastguard, police, ambulance services, air sea rescue and armed forces.

6. He must be able to take a good history and undertake and record a competent clinical examination.

7. He must be able to deliver first-aid and hygiene lectures to the crew and also conduct hygiene inspections and recognise occupational medical hazards. He should keep a watch for drug abuse.

8. He must maintain his sick bay in good order and make sure that an adequate supply of dressings, drugs and instruments is always available.

9. He must understand the necessity of delivering a good health care package to his barge, rig or platform.

10. He must maintain proper medical records for every person that he sees, however trivial the complaint.

11. He must also make sure that clear and well-laid-out reports are sent with medical evacuations.

12. He must be able to establish a satisfactory relationship with all those working on board the installation and especially with the barge captain, rig or platform manager.

13. He must be familiar with the regulations governing offshore medical standards.

In order to carry out these duties the rig medic will need to keep himself fit as he will have to climb about the platform and he may also have to transfer to a stand-by vessel or diving ship by winching or possibly by personnel basket. The medic will need to be examined to the same medical standard as all the other offshore workers.

It needs to be remembered that an offshore medic works very much in isolation, unlike a hospital nurse who is very much part of a medical team. The qualities required of a medic are rather different as he will not work a fixed schedule or have superiors or doctors available for ready consultation. At almost any offshore location anywhere in the world there is complete isolation and he needs to know that he can be self-sufficient and manage to cope. His nearest doctor may be a long way off and only contactable by radio.

A man or woman applying for such a job must be used to working away from home. Most of the medics normally operate on a rota and will be absent from the family in the same way as a merchant seaman or other offshore worker. There is no doubt that some families are not suited to this type of life.

A medic must be suited to the confined life on board a platform or barge. He should fit into a community life which is similar to being stationed at a small military or scientific outpost or even like being at boarding school! He needs to be able to organise his life offshore so that he can be on call for long hours and will need to arrange his surgery times to fit in with shift changes while he must also get accustomed to being disturbed during his sleeping hours. He needs to be able to establish a working relationship with his fellow employees so that while he must always be ready to discuss their problems in the sick bay he has to make sure that he is not troubled in the mess room. All these factors must be carefully studied before training a medic, and there is no doubt that adequate investigation of previous experience and family background may prevent unsuitable people being trained, thus saving time, unhappiness and money.

The medic should not be entirely preoccupied with the care of individuals, but should devote much attention to providing a good all round health service with emphasis on preventive medicine and positive health. It is important that he maintains a good relationship with the platform manager, which requires tolerance and understanding by both parties. The habit of the medic having a daily meeting with the platform manager is very useful, not only to discuss general medical matters, but also because the platform manager may say 'can you help Jones as he does not seem to be doing a very good job at the moment'. It could be that the medic already knows why Jones is not doing a particularly good job and can indicate to the platform manager that there are reasons. He clearly needs to be careful not to discuss or betray confidential information that a patient may have given him during the course of the consultation. The medic may indeed become the repository for many confidences during the course of consultations. He is fulfilling offshore the pastoral role of a general practitioner. A medic should not offer any advice about how a patient should cope with his anxieties, but his role as a listener is paramount.

The medic's responsibility must be to his barge captain or platform manager, and he should never forget that the latter is totally responsible for the installation and those on board. This is similar to a medical officer and his C.O. in the armed forces. He needs to visit regularly all parts of the installation (subject to the OIM's permission) and also keep an eye on safety procedures on work sites. He must consider the way in which he could evacuate casualties from any part of his installation and make sure that the first-aid equipment is readily available at work sites and in his sick bay.

The question of who employs a medic is very relevant to his position offshore. Most medics are employed by the offshore operator on the advice of their medical department. However, if the company has no medical department and does not wish to employ medics directly they can contract the work of supplying and training medics to another organisation which then selects and employs the medics and arranges routes of evacuation and the emergency doctors to be on call. They can also supply a doctor for regular medical inspections and assessment of the medics' work with a report to the operator. Some medics may prefer to be employed by such a company as they then feel part of a professional medical organisation able to offer impartial advice to the operator and it may even make the medic's professional position simpler if he and his patient do not have the same employer. Such organisations can provide a complete service, but this may be a more expensive way than their being employed by the operator. It may well be that a subcontracted medical service is a suitable way of employing medics where a relatively small number of medics are employed, while larger offshore operators can use such a company to select and train medics prior to employment.

A company supplying medics will not confine its activity to United Kingdom waters. Such companies will provide medics for anywhere in the world, while a medic can also be provided to accompany patients on journeys of any length. They will provide medics at sites in any remote locations or in support of other industrial projects or expeditions for scientific purposes. A company providing medics needs to be flexible to ensure that the services provided are exactly those required and at the right price. Medics appear to welcome changes of location from time to time as this may provide them with new opportunities and experiences.

Number and Type of Patients Seen by Medics

Figures from 1979 to 1982 suggested that a medic might see between 3% and 7% of the installation population per day. These statistics were obtained from both fixed installations and barges in the North Sea and further afield. However, more recent figures from 1984 gave an incidence of between 2% and 4%. The decrease in sickness rates may represent a more careful assessment of offshore workers prior to employment though it needs to be remembered that the offshore population is getting older. Of the cases seen, between 70% and 80% are new cases while the remainder are 'follow ups'. Less than 1% of persons employed offshore are evacuated per week for medical reasons. Most of these evacuations are carried on routine helicopter flights and it is unusual for special flights to be necessary. This reflects the fact that medics are normally able to contain and treat all but the most serious medical problems until a routine helicopter flight is available — thus saving money and emergency flying.

The approximate breakdown of cases seen by a group of offshore medics in the North Sea during the period 1982–1984 is as follows:

Medical cases	40%
Skin problems	10%
Musculoskeletal problems	5%–10%
Minor trauma	5%–10%
ENT problems	10%–15%
Eye problems	10%–15%

While medics normally supply regular returns of their workload, clearly the analysis of cases may vary substantially. The type of cases seen are in some ways similar to general practice, but it must be remembered that a GP devotes much of his time to children and geriatric problems and sees a very much wider range of problems. Some of the conditions which a medic treats offshore would not require the attention of a doctor onshore. This does not mean that this work is not necessary. The work of a medic offshore is most valuable and the very presence of a medic on board an installation should provide a great source of comfort to those offshore. The latter need the reassurance and availability of medics for many minor medical problems which would not require the presence of a doctor offshore. At present only one complex in the United Kingdom sector of the North Sea has a permanent medical officer on site, though occasionally special work such as some construction or diving may call for a resident offshore doctor.

Although it may appear that a medic may not be greatly occupied in seeing patients it should be remembered that medics are on duty 24 h per day and also have many other duties. Particularly important is their role in teaching first aid, maintaining their hospital and medical records, water testing, medical inspection of installations and lifeboats and attendance at safety meetings. Some medics on installations with a small population perform outside duties such as helicopter clerking and organising recreational activities, but these duties must always be secondary to their medical duties.

It must be remembered that the prime function of the medic is to provide skilled medical assistance in emergencies. It is important that an offshore medic establishes good relations with his supporting doctors onshore. These doctors are unlikely to be full-time occupational physicians and are probably groups of doctors (mainly GPs) retained for the specific purpose of supporting the offshore activities. The doctors should visit the offshore installation and the medics should visit the relevant medical establishments onshore. Medics should be encouraged to discuss their problems with their supporting doctors while these doctors should make sure that they inform offshore medics about the progress of personnel who have been evacuated. The North Sea Medical Centre in 1984–1985 had four or five calls per day from offshore medics seeking advice and it is very important that doctors are immediately available for such consultations, whether they come by radio or telephone. Good communications are the basis of good offshore medicine.

Selection and Training of Medics

At the time of going to press papers are circulating on this subject and new guidelines and legislation are likely in the near future. In the author's view all medics should be

SRNs, though it is possible that armed services SBAs might be acceptable. An SRN (now RGN) recruited from hospital as a medic should have several years' post-qualification experience as a charge nurse. In particular, he or she should have good experience in an accident and emergency department where in addition to casualties much 'run of the mill' general medical work, such as occurs in general practice, is seen. Medics should gain special experience in practical procedures such as putting up intravenous infusions, endotracheal intubation, resuscitation and catheterisation. Other areas in which a working knowledge is extremely helpful are opthalmology, ENT, dermatology, psychiatry and sexually transmitted diseases.

Above all the medic must be well versed in taking a full clinical history and performing a good clinical examination. He must develop his diagnostic skills and have a good knowledge of therapeutics. Prior to going offshore medics should undertake special training in diving medicine while they should also have experience of going under pressure. Courses in this subject are available at Aberdeen, Dundee and Great Yarmouth. The medic needs to have a good knowledge of the offshore health and safety regulations.

The Health and Safety Executive suggest at present that all medics should have a 4-week course before proceeding offshore and that they should be examined at the end of this course. A certificate should be granted and renewed every 3 years. It is also suggested that a refresher course of 2 weeks should be taken prior to re-certification. For first aiders it is suggested that a 5-day course should be taken prior to certification, which should be renewed again after a 1-day refresher course every 3 years. Certification and examination should be undertaken by doctors and others experienced in offshore medicine.

More extensive training for medics has been suggested with the possibility of a certificate or occupational health award for offshore medics. Such an award would add to the status of rig medics, improve morale and job satisfaction and also provide a specific identity and 'club' for medics. At present there is little doubt that medics are not well recognised as a group (particularly as they are often away from the United Kingdom) and a specific qualification would be helpful to them both individually and as a group. Those who are at present medics would need to be given adequate opportunity for training and certification before such regulations become mandatory.

Contractors' medics sometimes lack good supervision. A contractor may not possess a medical department and employ medics without making sure that they are well qualified and subject to assessment and surveillance, as would occur if they are employed through an operator's medical department or supplied by a reputable medic agency. There is also a tendency for such medics to be employed too much on non-medical duties. It is essential that contractors' medics are carefully supervised by doctors experienced in offshore medicine and not just placed on installations to satisfy the current regulations. It may be that offshore operators should ensure that their contractors provide efficient and well-supervised medics on the relevant installations. Rig medics should never be regarded as a legal necessity much of whose time can be devoted to non-medical duties, even though on installations with small numbers of personnel these medical duties may not be heavy. All contractors should make certain that their medics are supported by onshore doctors. It is useful that these retained doctors should exercise some supervision of the medic's work and visit the installation from time to time.

Medics and Diving

Medics may from time to time become involved with diving problems. In these cases, they should normally remain outside the chamber to support the diving supervisor, and to interpret and pass on to the shore doctor information being transmitted out of the chamber. It is unusual for the medic to have to enter the chamber, but there may be occasions when he is the only qualified person present to perform certain technical procedures such as setting up intravenous infusions or inserting catheters or endotracheal tubes.

All divers should be trained in first aid. The only person who may be at hand to save the life of a diver in trouble is his buddy. In addition to this there should always be at least one person in every saturation team who has had extra training in first aid and diving medicine, while in bounce diving (see p. 112), either air or mixed gas, a similar specially trained man should be available to enter a bell or compression chamber. Suggestions for the first aid and medical training of divers have been put forward by the European Undersea Biomedical Society while the Diving Medical Advisory Committee also issued a report in February 1983 discussing classes MTD(1) and MTD(2) (see Appendix 11).

Medical Facilities and Supplies

Most of the hospitals on drilling rigs and construction barges which the authors have inspected have clearly been designed without the benefit of any expert medical advice or even help from any of the experienced offshore medics. As a result they are functionally inefficient, inadequately equipped and badly laid out. For example, they usually have bunks, and too many, instead of free-standing beds. There are no work surfaces or washing facilities and very rarely is there any examination couch or operating table. The lighting is poor, the communications are so arranged that the medic has to leave his patient if he needs to speak to the doctor on shore, and he is usually expected to use the hospital as his own cabin. Rarely is there sufficient storage room for essential medical supplies.

In contrast, the hospitals on the recent generation of offshore production facilities, where oil company medical personnel have had an opportunity to advise the designers, are well suited to their function and reflect the expert thought which has gone into their design. It is hoped that the comments in this chapter will help to improve the design of future hospitals on drilling and construction contractors' equipment as well as helping the designers of production installations.

Some sort of first-aid facility is required on all manned offshore structures, no matter how many personnel there may be on board or how close it may be to the shore. Obviously the size and extent of the facility will depend upon the number of men it has to serve, and its location relative to the shore and other offshore medical units.

The layout and facilities of offshore sick bays are now defined in the Code of Practice to the Offshore Installations and Pipeline Works (First-Aid) Regulations (see Appendix 8). The main points specified are that the sick bay should be adequately heated, ventilated and lighted (with emergency lighting in addition); there shall be adequate electrical sockets and a wash basin with a constant supply of hot and cold water. The Code also specifies that there shall be flush toilets, a bath approachable from three sides, a shower and adequate working surfaces. It specifies

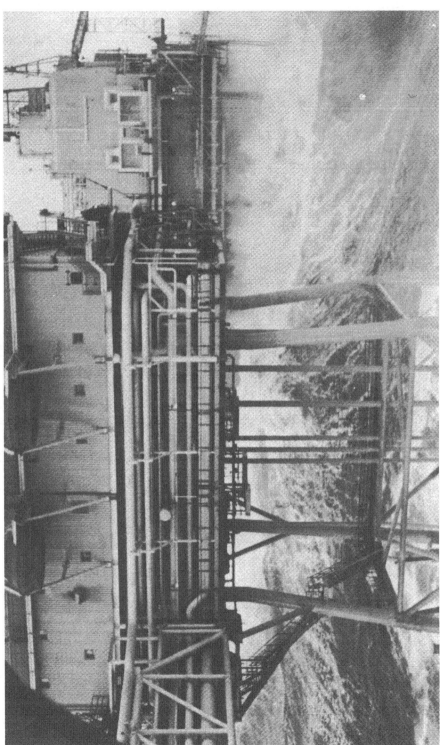

Fig. 5.1. Rough weather at Ekofisk.

the type of flooring and walls, the size of the doors and the siting of the sick bay in relation to the helipad and adjacent accommodation. It also forbids the use of the sick bay as quarters.

Even the smallest installations must have a first-aid room where a sick or injured man can be properly treated in privacy, and where a sick person can rest in bed. Any offshore unit may occasionally be isolated in bad weather, but it would be very unusual for an installation to be cut off for more than 48 h (Fig. 5.1). Any first-aid facility must be designed and equipped to accommodate a patient for this length of time. Even though first-aid facilities will be designed according to the number of men that are expected to be permanently resident on the installation, it must be remembered that additional personnel such as maintenance contractors are almost always on board and, in some cases, become a permanent feature of the installation.

Furthermore, the facilities must be designed and equipped so that they can be used as a reception area for casualties in the event of a disaster striking an adjacent rig (Fig. 5.2). The location of the hospital on the rig should be convenient for elevators and helideck, with as few corners and narrow passageways as possible for stretcher-bearing parties to negotiate.

The medical facilities should also be located close to a room, such as a mess room, lounge or recreation room, which can be quickly cleared of all furniture to provide a large open space for the performance of triage on a large number of casualties in a major disaster (Fig. 5.3). Collapsible beds of the 'camp bed' type can be provided and quickly erected when an influx of casualties is expected. Such space, provided by the recreation room in this case, was invaluable on the Ekofisk hotel at the time of the Alexander Kielland disaster.

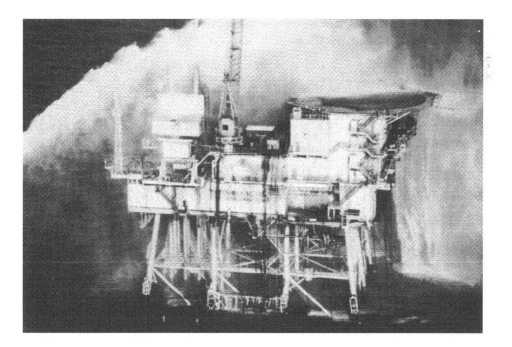

Fig. 5.2.   Ekofisk Bravo blowout, April 1977.

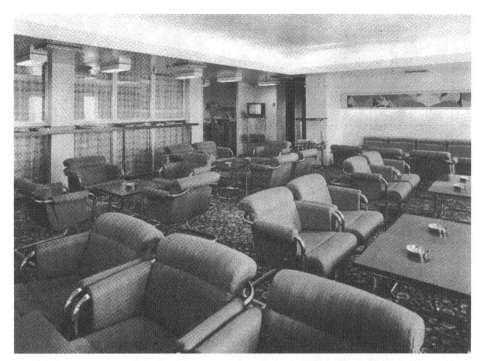

Fig. 5.3. One of the lounges at the Ekofisk hotel. Note the moveable furniture which can easily be cleared to provide a large open space for triage in the event of a major disaster.

Even the smallest facility, then, must have a room which can be designated the first-aid room, containing a single bed and big enough to take an additional fold-away bed when necessary. It should not be used as regular accommodation, but can be used as extra bed space in an emergency. It must have its own separate toilet and shower facilities. It must, in any case, contain a wash basin and it must have good lighting and an adequate working surface, and be well insulated against noise. On larger installations, there will need to be sick bay accommodation for up to six people in permanent, non-collapsible beds.

There are now several vessels operating in the North Sea which have been specially designed for fire fighting, diving, maintenance and general engineering. The S.S. Sedco-Phillips was one of the first and is illustrated in Fig. 5.4. One of the emergency functions of these vessels is to act as a reception station for large numbers of casualties in major incidents. They, therefore, have larger and more sophisticated hospitals (Fig. 5.5) with plenty of room for triage. In the event of fighting a fire they may have many casualties to deal with as part of their 'normal' work, quite apart from any they may receive during a 'disaster situation'. The level of training and competence of their medics as well as the equipping and stocking of their medical facilities must be commensurately higher than on conventional drilling or pipelaying equipment. They must be especially well stocked with all drugs, dressings, intra-venous fluids and other materials required for severe burns cases.

When the size of the first-aid room is not defined by legislation, it is recommended that the room is large enough to accommodate the requisite number of beds with at least 80 cm between each bed, which must be arranged in such a way that access is

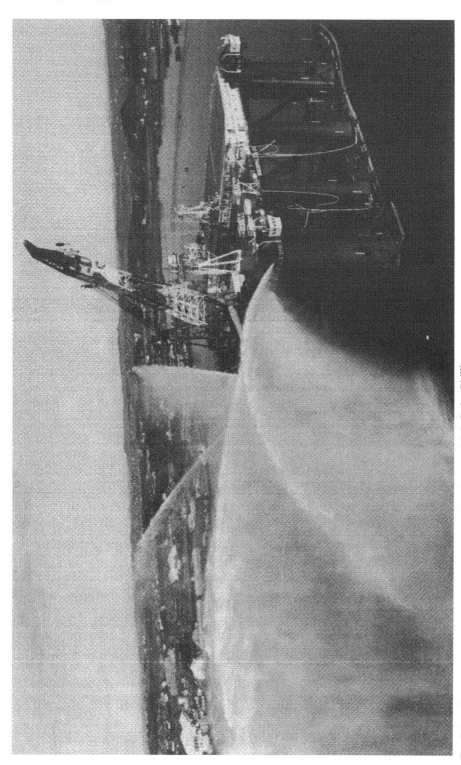

Fig. 5.4. The semisubmersible maintenance and fire fighting vessel S.S. Sedco-Phillips.

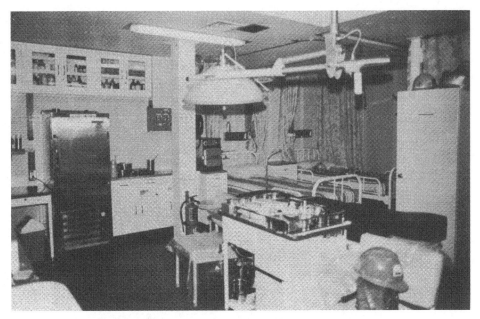

Fig. 5.5. A corner of the hospital on the S.S. Sedco-Phillips.

possible from all sides. In addition to the beds, the first-aid room must be large enough to accommodate the major items of equipment listed in Appendix 15.

It is an advantage to design the layout of the larger facilities in such a way that the beds can easily be separated to allow for the isolation of infectious or very seriously injured cases. Curtains must be provided around each bed so that they can be screened off when necessary.

The beds selected for the first-aid room should be of a standard hospital type, with rigid frames and base, and adjustable sections at head and foot to enable rapid change of the patient to a head-down position whichever way he is lying on the bed. At least one pair of cot sides should be kept on board for restraining a restless patient, and one lifting pole to enable patients to lift themselves up. The mattresses should be interior box-sprung, not foam rubber.

One bed and an examination couch are sufficient for installations with up to 100 persons on board. For numbers greater than this it may be necessary to provide one or more additional beds, but experience has shown that more than one bed is rarely required at any one time; however, under the new United Kingdom Offshore Installations and Pipeline Works (First-Aid) Regulations two beds are prescribed in the Appendix to the Guidance Notes for any installation with more than 26 persons on board.

The provision of oxygen and aspirator outlets is an advantage which saves a lot of space, but there are regulations restricting the provision of piped oxygen in offshore structures.

Except on the very smallest installations, where the first-aid room could be used as accommodation as long as it is not required for its proper purpose, the room should be kept exclusively for its designed purpose, and this is obligatory under Norwegian law. The medic or medics must be given their own quarters and they should not be expected to use the hospital beds as their own sleeping accommodation.

Somewhere on each rig, a free-standing bath for the immersion treatment of cases of hypothermia is required. Under Norwegian and British law this is mandatory. On larger installations this is most conveniently sited in the bathroom of the hospital but, on smaller rigs, it may be in one of the communal bathrooms or in the toolpusher's quarters. Wherever it is located, access to it must be possible from all sides so that the patient can be attended. Collapsible and canvas baths can be used to provide extra re-warming facilities in the event of there being a large number of hypothermic casualties.

In planning the first-aid room or hospital, allowance should be made for an adequate number of electric points. Many electrical appliances may be in use simultaneously — portable lights, aspirator, refrigerator, autoclave and various instruments which require electrical power. The floor should be tiled and sloped towards a central draining point for easy cleaning. There should be two sinks with elbow lever mixer taps — one for dirty jobs and the other for 'scrubbing up'.

There will need to be an adjustable minor operating table with a shadowless light over it. Other specialised furniture needed will be storage cupboards for drugs and dressings, including: a small double-locked cupboard for scheduled drugs; a small refrigerator for the storage of vaccines, blood specimens and some drugs; a steriliser and small autoclave; an adjustable desk light and a dressing trolley.

There should be double doors to the hospital with a total width not less than 120 cm, so that a stretcher party (two men on either side of a stretcher) can enter easily.

In planning the rig hospital it must be remembered that the facilities may need to be used in an emergency by a mobile surgical or intensive care team (see Chap. 4). The hospital may also be required for the performance of intensive resuscitation on severely injured personnel, and even emergency surgery. There must therefore be plenty of space, good lighting (not necessarily natural daylight) and enough storage room to hold the large amounts of emergency supplies which are required, such as stretchers, collapsible beds, blankets, intravenous fluids, and large dressings, which are needed in a disaster situation.

Waste disposal from the first-aid room can be a problem. Blood- or pus-soaked dressings, and disposable needles and syringes cannot be put in the usual waste bags for transportation ashore. Needles can be cut into two or three pieces to avoid their re-use and then discarded. Syringes and soiled dressings are best incinerated. With the increasing employment of women offshore, incinerators for the disposal of sanitary towels are required and these are also suitable for burning soiled dressings. Disposable sanitary towels and tampons tend to block the drains when flushed down the toilets on offshore platforms because the fall-away is not steep enough. Where incinerators are not available, soiled dressings, tampons and sanitary towels should be sealed in heavy-duty polythene bags and burned offshore or buried onshore.

There must be an intercom system for the medic between the hospital, his cabin and the radio room or control room. There should also be a telephone extension in the hospital from the rig-to-shore telephone communications system, so that the medic can speak directly to the shore doctor without leaving the patient.

There should be some provision on every installation for the temporary accommodation of a body. Unfortunately the time is bound to arise when a body, perhaps as the result of an accident, must be retained on board either while investigators arrive on the scene or until transport ashore is available. It is understandably distasteful for the rest of the crew to have the body of one of their colleagues in a cabin or lying in a passageway. A well-ventilated compartment or box big enough to hold a corpse is all that is required. It should be sited on the outside of the rig, and on some installations the space is often normally used for the storage of vegetables (see also p. 144). During storage, bodies are best contained in heavy-duty polythene bags with a full-length zipper. These are fluid and odour tight and are fitted with carrying handles. At least two should be kept on every installation.

Stretchers

Stretchers for use offshore must secure the patient in such a way that he can be rescued from cramped and inaccessible situations, transported along narrow, steep passageways and staircases over water, and manoeuvred easily in and out of helicopters. In addition, the stretcher should allow easy access to the patient for examination purposes, both offshore and when he reaches the hospital. The litter type of stretcher is difficult to handle, prevents proper examination of the patient and does not permit X-rays to be taken while the patient is in it. Furthermore, the wire mesh of the metal types tends to break, and sharp ends can be dangerous to the patient and attendants as well as tearing the upholstery of ambulances. The use of glass fibre has eliminated some of these disadvantages but, in spite of their popularity with some safety officers, they are not very suitable for use in the offshore situation. The Neil-Robertson fabric and cane stretcher is a traditional and effective type of stretcher for use at sea, which can be lifted by a crane or helicopter winch in a horizontal position. The Paraguard stretcher, developed from the Neil-Robertson but made of telescopic tubular steel and PVC, is a great improvement and is ideally suited to the offshore situation. It is light, durable, collapsible, but rigid when assembled, and it can be slung in a horizontal position with the patient tightly secured.

There are various other types of stretchers such as the MFC Powell inflatable stretcher, the Laerdal vacuum mattress stretcher and the Kennion-Irvine industrial rescue stretcher. These stretchers all claim to have varying advantages, but in most cases they are more bulky to store and take up more space in a helicopter when accommodating a patient, and in some cases are more complicated to assemble and use. In the opinion of the authors, none of them has advantages which outweigh the simplicity and convenience of the Paraguard stretcher in the offshore situation.

Mechanial Aids to Respiration

Though mouth-to-mouth artificial respiration and external cardiac compression must be the primary means of maintaining life when cardiopulmonary arrest occurs for any reason, there is a requirement for a mechanical means of ventilation if only to take the strain off the operator. Mouth-to-mouth artificial respiration is a very exhausting procedure. If positive pressure artificial respiration has to be maintained during a journey then a mechanical means of administering it is essential.

There is a bewildering variety of mechanical respirators on the market, but only three which satisfy the currently recommended international standards are available in Britain. The minimum standards for an oxygen-powered automatic ventilator are: (a) It should be manually triggered; (b) it should give a minimum flow rate of 100 l oxygen per minute; and (c) It should deliver oxygen at 100% concentration.

To achieve these minimum standards, the machine must be volume-cycled and not pressure-cycled. The subject was reviewed by Harries (1979). The PACE SOS resuscitator, now marketed by AMBU International, is very simple to use and has proved very reliable under field conditions.

In the past there has been some reluctance on the part of the first-aid training organisations to advocate the general administration of oxygen in cases of hypoxia on the grounds that it may induce apnoea in chronic bronchitics. However, the consensus of opinion is now in favour of using 100% oxygen wherever ventilation is inadequate as it is considered that its undoubted benefit far outweighs the largely hypothetical risk associated with its administration to some bronchitics.

To provide adequate inflation of the lungs, the face mask of any respirator must be applied to the face with an air-tight fit, and the airway should be maintained through the insertion of a Guerdel airway.

Aspirators powered by compressed air or oxygen are not powerful enough to remove any semi-solid material, such as regurgitated stomach contents, from the pharynx. Such material must either be removed by hand or using an electrically operated or foot-operated suction pump, one of which should be kept in every offshore first-aid room.

Instruments, Drugs and Dressings

The medical supplies on any rig must be commensurate with the training and capability of the medics, and with their increasing competence there is a requirement for increasingly sophisticated equipment. It has been suggested, for example, that offshore hospitals should have X-ray and electrocardiograph facilities. It is the opinion of the authors that this type of equipment is not needed; if it were provided, it would raise medico-legal problems in the interpretation of films or tracings. Medics, however well trained or experienced, are not qualified to accept the responsibility of interpreting X-rays or ECGs, and no shore-based doctor is going to delegate such responsibilities to them. Furthermore, any patient whose symptoms appear to require an X-ray or an ECG to establish a diagnosis should be sent ashore for proper assessment. An X-ray or ECG, taken offshore in the absence of a qualified doctor, is unlikely to resolve the situation and would certainly not help a doctor onshore to decide that a patient is fit to remain on the rig. Such sophisticated diagnostic apparatus would of course have a place on an installation where a doctor is resident, or where accurate pictures can be sent ashore by slow scan television; there is also a strong case for using computerised ECG machines from which tracings can be transmitted directly to the doctor onshore over the normal telephone system.

It is essential, however, to supply the medics with enough instruments and equipment for them to fulfil their duties. These include stethoscope, sphygmomanometer, eye-testing chart, diagnostic set (auriscope and ophthalmoscope), scalpel, forceps, artery forceps, needle holders, suture materials, etc. A list of suggested equipment appears in Appendix 1.

Inflatable splints should be supplied and adequate quantities of bandages and dressings, especially large shell dressings and Roehampton burn dressings. Tube gauze and appropriate applicators are more convenient to use than cotton bandages.

There is a tendency to overstock with drugs. Relatively small quantities are required, except of such items as soluble aspirin, cough linctuses and throat lozenges. A variety of essential drugs which will enable the onshore doctor to prescribe appropriately for any condition include analgesics, antispasmodics, antihistamines, antibiotics, hypnotics, gastrointestinal sedatives, tranquillisers, resuscitative agents such as hydrocortisone and various dermatological and ophthalmic preparations, including Parolein eye drops for removing oil from the eyes.

The question of analgesics is often raised, as there seems to be some reluctance to hold supplies of opiates offshore in the British sector. Such supplies can be held under the jurisdiction of the onshore doctor, as long as a Controlled Drugs Register is kept and the drugs are stored in a double-locked cabinet in accordance with the Controlled Drugs Regulations. In the opinion of the authors, it is essential that a badly injured person is made comfortable by the administration of the appropriate dose of analgesics before he is subjected to the discomfort of a long helicopter flight, and opiates are still the best analgesics to use except where they are specifically contraindicated. Pentazocine may be a reasonable alternative, but only when it is administered parenterally in adequate dosage. It may cause hallucinations and disorientation.

If anaesthesia is required, local or regional blocks should be used, so adequate supplies of lignocaine should be stocked. If a general anaesthetic has to be given for some reason, then an anaesthetist with appropriate equipment should be flown out. In the most extreme circumstances, if a general anaesthetic must be given and it is not possible to get a specialist anaesthetist, then ketamine administered through the intravenous line is probably the safest and most effective method, as long as an efficient aspirator and an airway are to hand.

The list of drugs which are required to be held on board British installations appears in Appendix 1. Larger quantities of specialised equipment and drugs which may be needed if a rig or platform receives a large number of casualties from an adjacent disaster area must be held and stored separately from the regular items. A list of such additional supplies can be found in Appendix 4.

Survival Suits

Whether or not to provide passengers in helicopters with survival suits for protection from immersion hypothermia in the event of a crash is a vexed and much-debated question. On the one side are those that maintain that the chances of one's survival in the sea are greatly improved if a suit is worn which insulates the wearer against the cold. Protagonists of this argument would also maintain that an unspecified number of people who have been involved in helicopter crashes in the North Sea would have survived if they had been wearing survival suits, and that the risks of such a crash occurring justify the cost and inconvenience of providing such clothing.

The antagonists, on the other hand, argue against survival suits, not on the grounds of cost, but on the grounds that they are unnecessary. They point out that the dangers of flying by helicopter are no greater than in a scheduled aircraft, and would support their contention by citing helicopter services over water, such as from Penzance to the Scilly Isles, where passengers are not expected to wear survival suits. They would also contend that immersion suits are only a second best aid to survival, which is best ensured by enabling the passengers to transfer from the aircraft to a covered life raft as quickly as possible. The antagonists would also maintain that the very wearing of survival suits raises passenger anxiety and gives a misleading impression that helicopter flying is full of danger. Some helicopter pilots, in the United Kingdom sector of the North Sea at least, apparently have more confidence in themselves and their machines, as indicated by their steadfast refusal to wear survival suits. There is no denying that survival suits are also inconvenient and uncomfortable for the wearers, and at times have even produced dangerous hyperthermia. Most wearers will admit to being unhappy at the threat to personal hygiene from wearing other people's cast-off survival suits. Admittedly this problem can be obviated by the issue of personal suits, but this is not practical in most situations where offshore crews and subcontractors are constantly changing. It is unpleasant to put your feet into a survival suit in which the previous occupant has left a sample of his urine, as has happened on more than one occasion.

No matter which argument may be correct, the subject has passed from the medical or scientific arena to the political. Once one company had decided that its helicopter passengers should wear survival suits, the others felt they must do likewise in case they could be publicly and unfavourably compared in the event of a fatal accident. After that, legislative bodies have either persuaded, or compelled (as in Norway) all companies to adopt a mandatory policy regarding the wearing of immersion suits by passengers flying by helicopter over the sea.

Since there is such disagreement about the very necessity for wearing survival suits, it is hardly surprising that there is no standard design and a bewildering variety of alternative choices, each commercially promoted by the manufacturers with little regard for the requirements or convenience of the wearers, or the scientific validity of the tests upon which their claims are made.

In an endeavour to enable scientific comparisons to be made between the different models, so that choice could be based on objective assessment and not commercial advantage, various authors have considered this complex subject, and an attempt made to establish objective standards for survival suits by Leese and Norman in 1979.

The UKOAA Medical Advisory Committee produced a report in 1978 which defined 'a basic specification for the design and evaluation of survival suits'. The main features of that report were as follows:

1. Any survival suit is only to be regarded as one aid in transferring a survivor of a ditched helicopter to a survival craft. The aim should be to ensure that the survivor is kept dry and warm during the transfer, and the provision of a survival suit is only one part of the overall operation and should not be regarded as an end in itself.

2. The survival suit must keep the survivor dry, or almost dry, when he is submerged up to his neck in water.

3. The suit when worn over ordinary clothing should not allow a fall of core body temperature of more than 2°C after 2 h immersion in water at 5°C.

4. The suit must be of single-piece design.

5. It must provide cover for the head.

6. Mittens should be provided as separate but attached items.

7. The suit should have feet or boots as an integral part of it.

8. The suit should be designed to be worn over normal clothing.

9. The suit must be constructed in such a way that it is easy to get in and out of.

10. The suit must be hard-wearing and easily cleaned.

11. The suit must be made of non-flammable material.

12. The suit must be made in such a way that it can be adequately ventilated when worn in the summer to avoid over-heating.

13. The suit must not allow air-trapping.

14. The suit should be constructed of a material of a conspicuous luminous colour.

15. No attempt should be made to incorporate buoyancy in the suit. Buoyancy aids should be separately provided.

16. The suits can either be manufactured to fit individual personnel or in a broad range of sizes which permit interchange between different personnel.
17. The suits must be worn on every helicopter flight, although it may be reasonable to dispense with them when the water temperature is higher than 15°C and the air temperature higher than 21°C.
18. A survival suit cannot function as a working suit, and no attempt should be made to combine the two functions in a single garment.
19. The suit must be sufficiently comfortable that it is totally acceptable to the wearer.

In any situation where immersion is a threat to life, the best means of ensuring survival is to get from the water into a dry floating device such as an inflatable dinghy, which should be covered in extreme conditions of either heat or cold. No matter what protective clothing is worn, immersion is likely to result in death from hypothermia or drowning in a relatively short time, compared with the relatively long survival which can be expected once the victim is out of the water. Even if hypothermia is prevented, drowning will occur from the inhalation of sea water from even moderate seas unless the victim's face is protected by some sort of visor. The Civil Aviation Authority have now instructed that spray hoods should be an integral part of life jackets worn by helicopter passengers. It would seem prudent, therefore, to devise better means of ensuring that in a helicopter accident the life rafts are launched and survivors can transfer to them as quickly as possible, even if they get wet in the process.

As was stated in an editorial of the British Medical Journal in December 1978,

> We must, however, be aware of over-emphasising the value of protective suits in promoting survival. When a helicopter makes a forced landing on the water, for example, the passengers who escape serious injury on impact will be almost guaranteed survival if they could be transferred, with or without survival suits, to a dry, covered inflatable dinghy. Yet in some of the helicopter accidents in the North Sea in the past 12 years deaths from hypothermia or drowning have occurred because the occupants have been unable to reach life rafts. If we are to prevent such deaths the ideal of transferring survivors to a dry, covered life raft demands solutions to many problems — including the stability and flotation of the helicopters; where to place the rafts (possibly on the outside of the machine); and training crews in methods of escaping from a stricken helicopter and in the techniques of self preservation. Immersion suits are certainly important, but in the past they have been considered an easy solution — distracting attention from the wider and more important aspects of preventing immersion hypothermia and drowning.

For a review of the current concepts concerning survival after helicopter ditching and the use of immersion suits, the reader is referred to the report of a workshop held at the Royal College of Physicians (UKOOA-IAUMED 1984). This workshop was comprised of representatives of the oil industry, helicopter operators, academic institutions and rescue services and it considered the requirement for immersion suits, the physiological basis for survival policy, the specification of immersion suit performance and the design, construction and testing of immersion suits. Its conclusions should be required reading for all those people who have responsibility for determining policies regarding the wearing of survival suits as well as their design and construction (obtainable from UKOOA Ltd., 3 Hans Crescent, London SW1X 0LN).

Communications and Transport

Good clear channels of communication are a vital part of any offshore project, and they are particularly vital in the management of medical problems.

There are various communication routes available:

1. By radio-telephone link with the public telephone service and the local coastal radio station
2. By the company's radio-telephone link between its local office and the offshore installation
3. By a tropospheric scatter link between the offshore rig and a central communications centre, operated by the company onshore
4. By a direct radio-telephone line between the doctor's office and the offshore installation
5. By a telex link, which may be a private service belonging to the company or part of the public international telex system

In addition to the above, there are of course, radio and possibly radio-telex links between the installations themselves, and also radio links between the helicopter base and the platform. Finally, the local coastguard station will have an offshore radio-telephone link. Any, or all, of the channels may well be needed in a major emergency, but none of them are really suitable for the daily communications needed between the doctors onshore and the crews on the rig.

The communications route chosen for the location will depend upon local circumstances but, if onshore back-up medical services are to function efficiently and quickly, the link to the doctor must be direct and clear.

The offshore medic is the eyes, ears and hands of the onshore doctor, and he must be able to talk directly to the doctor from the side of the patient. That means that there must be a direct telephone link from the hospital on the rig, so that the medic does not have to leave the patient and go to the radio room, or have to relay messages through the radio room.

The duty doctor onshore must be easily and quickly contactable, and usually requires that each member of the onshore medical team is supplied with some sort of radio-pager. There is now a plethora of communications devices available ranging from simple bleeping systems to mobile hand-held telephones. In practice, a system allowing two-way communication is the most useful for a doctor on call.

The most difficult time for maintaining communications is during transit of the doctor between the shore and a rig. During this period, messages have to be passed between the rig's radio room, air traffic control, and the helicopter pilot, with inevitable distortion. Personal radios are of little help in these circumstances. The best solution is for the second-on-call back-up doctor onshore to maintain liaison with the rig until such time as the first doctor arrives.

The quality of modern radio communications is so good that it is unusual to experience any significant disruption or distortion. However, in times of major disasters or crises, all normal radio and telephone channels may be blocked by other calls and, in these circumstances, an emergency telephone line — a 'hot line' as it were — may be invaluable. Such a line might link the offices of the operating companies with the police headquarters, the helicopter air traffic control room, the doctor's office, and perhaps the local coastguard headquarters. In a circuit such as this, any member whose normal outside lines are blocked can establish a communication route via one of the others, at the expense of less confidentiality — but that is insignificant in these sorts of circumstances.

One of the problems of radio communications is that there is no standardisation of channels. For example in an emergency, helicopters may not be able to communicate with lifeboats except via their base and the coastguard. Communications through a third, or even a fourth party, such as the helicopter control room, the oil company base, or the coastguard, inevitably become distorted, especially in emergency conditions. Every effort should be made, therefore, to maintain communications links as direct as possible, with the avoidance of intermediaries.

Telex, although slightly slower, is accurate and produces an immediate, permanent record of the conversation. A telex machine should certainly be a standard piece of equipment in the office of any group of doctors providing emergency cover for the oil industry.

The Diving Medical Advisory Committee has compiled an *aide-mémoire* for use by medics and doctors in the management of diving emergencies. This enables an offshore medic or diving emergency medical technician to gather all relevant information about the problem before he contacts the doctor onshore, who also has a copy of the blank form. Whether contact is by radio or telex, therefore, the medic should be able to transmit his answers to the various questions in such a way that the doctor will eventually have a duplicate copy giving him a full picture of the situation. This not only reduces opportunities for error but also provides a permanent record of the incident for future reference. The form is designed in such a way that the majority of answers can be indicated by marking an appropriate box. A copy of this *aide-mémoire* is included in Appendix 12.

The communications centre at the doctor's office is absolutely vital. Automatic answering devices have no place in communications systems for offshore medical care. All communications, telephone, radio and telex should come to a central manned point, where there should be an operator constantly during normal working hours. There are various systems available for the transferring of calls during the quiet hours but, whatever system is chosen, the caller must get straight through to the duty doctor without having to make two or three calls. Again, recorded messages or calls interrupted to be transferred to another number are time-wasting and annoying to the caller. Furthermore, if the call is coming from an offshore installation or a ship, it may have taken some time to establish and the link may well be lost in trying to re-establish the connection.

Transport of personnel, mail and some light goods is by helicopter in most cases. In all cases of medical emergency, the speed, versatility and comfort of helicopters will ensure that they will remain the primary means of moving casualties.

Most helicopters can be quickly fitted with winches when it is necessary to transfer someone to or from a vessel which has no landing facilities. Some operators keep a helicopter permanently in the field with the winch already fitted. It takes about 15 min to fit one to a machine when required and, as having a winch permanently fitted reduces the helicopter's payload, other companies elect to have the apparatus available for fitting to whichever machine happens to be available at the time.

Workboats are used for the conveyance of supplies and materials. These boats are usually of about 1000 tons size, with large open decks aft of the accommodation and wheel house, which is set well forward. The open deck facilitates the stowage of drillpipe, and makes loading and unloading much easier alongside a rig where the vessel cannot tie up, but has to maintain its position by the use of its main engines and thrusters, and the cargo has to be lifted 60 ft or more to the deck of the rig by crane (Fig. 1.19).

There are also stand-by boats at every rig. These are usually old trawlers, though specially designed rescue boats with accommodation for 300 people have been introduced recently. Stand-by boats are solely for use in emergencies, when they may be called upon to help in the evacuation of a rig or to pick up people who may have fallen into the sea, or survivors who have abandoned a stricken installation. Since this is their role, it would certainly be sensible to design the boats accordingly, with adequate facilities for the resuscitation and treatment of casualties, the accommodation of a large number of survivors and suitable means of easily picking survivors out of the sea. It is also necessary that their crews should be properly trained in rescue and first aid.

Transporting a Sick or Injured Person

Normally a sick or injured man will be brought ashore by helicopter but, occasionally, weather conditions may prevent this or cause long delays. In such circumstances an alternative means such as a supply boat, workboat or stand-by boat will have to be considered. However, transport by ship is likely to take a long time, and transfer from the rig to the vessel can be hazardous in bad weather conditions. On the other hand, there is more room on a ship and conditions may be rather more comfortable for the patient.

Weather conditions may make flying hazardous, but helicopter crews will often be prepared 'to have a go' in bad weather in order to bring help to a fellow worker in trouble. In these conditions, the doctor has an additional factor to consider in deciding on the urgency and method of medical evacuation, because of the potential danger to the helicopter crew and, possibly, himself if he is to go and 'collect' the casualty.

All these factors have to be taken into account when the doctor and the medic are deciding on the requirement for a 'casevac'. On the one hand, some cases, such as severe burns, need to be brought ashore as quickly as possible, but on the other, there is nothing more annoying to the helicopter crews and embarrassing to the doctor than a supposedly badly injured man who walks off the helicopter with his finger in a bandage after a hazardous emergency flight. Many emergencies may appear to be much more urgent to the attendants offshore than they do to the experienced doctor onshore, but he must also realise that he has a duty to relieve their anxiety, either by giving clear instructions and reassurance, or by having the casualty evacuated. These can be some of the most difficult decisions that the back-up doctor is called upon to make.

Occasionally, in a ship-borne evacuation, time can be saved if the doctor goes out in the local lifeboat to rendezvous with the casualty vessel, but usually these are the only circumstances in which the local lifeboat service can be of any real assistance in offshore emergency situations.

Whatever means of transport is chosen, it is vitally important that the patient should be resuscitated and his condition stabilised before the journey is commenced. Managing a desperately ill or shocked person in either an aircraft or a ship is extremely difficult, and may well result in the death of the patient. Shock must be countered by the administration of intravenous fluids such as plasma expanders or plasma itself before the journey is started. The intravenous line should be left open throughout the journey, and in many cases which may not be suffering from established shock, a precautionary intravenous line may prove extremely valuable. There should never be any hesitation in putting one up, even though it may sometimes prove to have been unnecessary. Other drugs such as hydrocortisone and vasopressors may be administered as needed, and adequate analgesia should be induced before the patient's journey begins. Choice of analgesic will depend to some extent upon personal preference, but adequate doses of opiate are the most effective, and only contraindicated where there may be respiratory depression.

The patient may either be accompanied ashore by the medic, or the duty doctor may go out to return with the casualty. In either case the attendant must ensure that all the equipment, including a mechanical resuscitator, drugs, intravenous fluids, instruments, dressings, and other items are on the aircraft or ship before departure. An emergency check list would include:

Burns dressings
Hydrocortisone
Morphine
Macrodex or dextran
Flynn resuscitator
Syringes and needles
Artery forceps
Intravenous-giving sets
Metaraminol
Portable aspirator
Ryle's tube
Foley catheter
Endotracheal tube and laryngoscope or oesophageal obturator airway

Finally, on arrival ashore the helicopter should land, if possible, at the local hospital. The less handling a shocked patient is subjected to the better, and transfer from helicopter to hospital by ambulance should therefore be avoided if at all possible. All hospitals which may have to receive casualties from an offshore operation should have facilities for a helicopter to land, and when a new operation is set up, an early visit should be made to the local hospital by the chief pilot, accompanied by the emergency doctor, to survey the facilities, establish the precise location, flight path for approach, persons to contact, availability of night landing facilities, etc. Where there are no landing facilities at the hospital, there may be no alternative but to land on a suitable piece of open ground conveniently close, and transport the patient the last part of the journey by ambulance. In these circumstances it will be necessary to have a written procedure in conjunction with the local police, fire and ambulance services, all of which will be involved.

Stand-by Vessels

This section is based in the main on observations and experience in the United Kingdom sector of the North Sea. The regulations quoted are British, and if the medical problems of stand-by vessels in other areas are being considered, the appropriate government rules must be taken into account. Much useful information is contained in the Department of Transport Instructions for the Guidance of Surveyors 1984.

The Offshore Installations Regulations 1976 (SI 1976 No. 1542) state that it is necessary for there to be a stand-by vessel within 5 nautical miles of every offshore installation when it is manned. This requirement applies to both fixed and mobile installations. The main functions of such a stand-by vessel are:

1. To assist in the rescue of installation personnel during an emergency
2. To accommodate installation personnel on a short-term basis in the event of a total evacuation
3. To provide first aid to rescued personnel
4. To act as a radio station able to communicate with the installation being covered, with other vessels and installations in the vicinity, and with coastal radio stations
5. To rescue any person in the water near the installation
6. To provide close attendance upon the relevant installations, and to be fully prepared to rescue persons during the following operations: (a) helicopter landing and take-off; (b) personnel working over the side and near the water

The most important role of the stand-by vessels is in providing life-saving cover for personnel on offshore installations in time of an emergency. They might be better designated rescue rather than stand-by vessels. It should not be assumed that stand-by vessels are automatically the best way of supporting installations in emergencies. It could be argued that the installation itself should be responsible for its own rescue facilities, though undoubtedly in the United Kingdom sector of the North Sea stand-by vessels will remain. The arguments are well presented in a report to the Department of Energy in 1981.

Stand-by vessels are mainly converted deep or mid-water side trawlers which are seaworthy and versatile. While, however, they may be excellent for major emergencies such as a total rig evacuation, in the more likely single man overboard incident or helicopter ditching, their speed and manoeuvrability may not be suitable for a rapid response. In the latter situation rigid inflatables are much more likely to be useful. These should be seaworthy in open conditions with winds of up to gale force. They should provide a safe working platform for their crews, have a speed up to 30 knots and have a low freeboard for recovery of survivors. They must be able to be rapidly launched and one member of the crew should be permanently dressed ready. Emergency medical equipment needs to be carried in these vessels and the following are suggested:

1. Triangular bandages and dressings
2. 3-in. Adhesive plaster and crepe bandages
3. Scissors and safety pins
4. Laerdal face mask and Guerdel airway(s)
5. Protective waterproof sheets
6. Stretchers capable of being lifted onto the mother ship or by helicopter
7. Powerful searchlight

It is essential that the equipment (bar the stretcher) is carried in waterproof containers and the contents are frequently checked to make sure that they remain useable.

The stand-by vessel itself requires accommodation to receive in an emergency all the personnel on board the installation for which it is responsible.

This does not mean that a sophisticated hospital is necessary as 90% of those rescued should constitute 'walking wounded' and be accommodated in areas where there is plenty of seating: 10% allowance should be made for those who will need to lie down in special bunks and space must be available for a few to undergo intensive care. Stand-by vessels are not in general meant to provide long-stay accommodation for seriously ill or injured personnel. It is essential that space should be provided for their initial resuscitation, but after this they should be transferred probably by helicopter to land or an installation hospital, or put ashore when the ship reaches port. It is important that if a large number of casualties are taken aboard the stand-by vessel, a member of the crew should be responsible for sorting out those casualties who need immediate care and attention. Triage ideally should take place as close as possible to exit from the water, but unfortunately the design of some stand-by vessels means a considerable distance has to be travelled to the sorting area and this may involve some vertical climbing. Some larger stand-by vessels now carry service-trained medical personnel who could manage the triage if they are not occupied with seriously ill patients.

It is very important that adequate space is provided for the reception of casualties. Bunks and/or seats should be provided in adequate amounts so that not more than 10% of the survivor capacity is accounted for as standing. Attention should be devoted to seeing that heating, lighting, ventilation and access to reception areas are satisfactory. Baths (collapsible or fixed) need to be provided for the treatment of hypothermia. An intensive care area is needed where resuscitation, transfusion, splinting and arrest of haemorrhage can be carried out on suitable tables. Ship-to-shore communications should be available in this area.

A stand-by vessel must be equipped with ladders and scrambling nets. It should also be possible to provide a 'floating depot' for survivors to get into, before they are lifted onto the stand-by vessel. Some thought should be devoted to the method by which seamen are rescued from the sea and consideration given as to whether people should be allowed to climb any great vertical height. Special attention needs to be devoted to lifting casualties, particularly the middle-aged, who have been in the water for a prolonged period. It is preferable to lift them from the water in a position as near horizontal as possible.

This may be possible by the use of self-draining stretchers, ladders or special strops. The rigid inflatable may be particularly useful in lifting casualties from the sea in the first place by virtue of its low freeboard and it can be used as a stretcher, but there still remains the problem of getting the casualties out of the inflatable. Most stand-by vessels have special openings in their gunwales to provide for a short climb from the sea to the deck, though in heavy weather large quantities of water may be shipped. It is only possible to haul survivors over about 1 m freeboard.

All stand-by vessels should be provided with a suitable place for winching to and from a helicopter. This area needs good lighting and a landing area clear of mast and aerials. Casualties can be transferred to a helicopter either on stretchers or by an ordinary winching lift. Although this facility is not available on all stand-by vessels (particularly in the southern sector of the North Sea) it should be a regular feature as it may be dangerous or impossible to raise and lower people without an adequately clear space, particularly in bad weather. Not only may it be necessary to evacuate casualties, but it may be necessary to lower a doctor or medic on board a stand-by vessel. If it is impossible to lift somebody onto a helicopter from the stand-by vessel then it is also likely to be difficult to lift them off by any other means, for example, personnel basket.

Medical Selection of Crew

The selection of crew members for a stand-by vessel is of major importance and they must be subjected to full and careful medical examination. The examination should be repeated at regular intervals not greater than every 2 years until the age of 35 years, and annually following this. It is also desirable that a member of the crew should be re-examined if he is absent from work for 14 or more consecutive days through illness or injury. Crew members should be examined by a doctor who is fully conversant with the rigorous conditions under which these stand-by vessels operate.

It should be realised that a man may be on a vessel for 28 days at a time, and that conditions in the North Sea are particularly exacting in winter. Anyone who has seen a stand-by vessel pitching and tossing in a force eight gale will understand the problems that these men face. The crew members must be suitable for long periods of rather repetitive duties, interspersed with sudden periods of intense physical activity. The length of the voyage may vary from 21 to 28 days and it should not be more than the latter figure, though occasionally voyages up to 35 days have been served. Such a short voyage may seem attractive to people on foreign-going ships, but it should be borne in mind that voyages in the North Sea on small vessels can be extremely arduous and very cold. There is little doubt that physical and mental fitness on board a stand-by vessel is of paramount importance. The medical examination should be carried out by a doctor approved under the Merchant Shipping (Medical Examination) Regulations 1983 (SI 1983 No. 808) and the standards should be those laid down in Merchant Shipping Notice M.1144. In the author's view, it is not satisfactory to have the medical examinations performed by the crewman's own GP. The examination should be performed by an independently retained doctor, who has no personal interest in a particular patient obtaining a job. The doctor has to assess the seaman's working capacity in relation to the physical and mental requirements of the work. During the course of the examination he should consider not only the interests of the employer in finding a suitable employee, but also whether the individual is suited to and safe for the job.

It is understandable that most GPs will feel bound to try to do their best to provide their own patients with employment, but this may be in the interests of neither the employee nor the employer. No departure from the highest standards of both physical and mental health is justified, and passing anybody as fit who is not strictly up to the standards laid down by a particular company or its medical advisers nearly always leads to subsequent difficulties. In performing the crew member's examination it is important to review the previous medical history to assess his suitability for offshore work and its attendant problems. The potential employee should fill in a form giving his previous medical history and on this form he should sign to say that he has given a true account and also consents to a report about his health being given to his potential employers.

In the course of the examination, particular attention should be paid to obesity and to any orthopaedic defect which might give rise to difficulty in standing on the deck of a pitching vessel. Particular attention should also be paid to personal cleanliness of cooks and stewards who should also have stool examinations. The Norwegian regulations require all seafarers to be tested audiometrically and the same policy should apply to the crews of stand-by and supply vessels of all nationalities as it is the only legally satisfactory way of assessing hearing. The importance of wearing ear protectors in engine rooms and other noisy areas should be stressed. At the conclusion of the examination the potential employer should be issued with a certificate indicating that the candidate has been examined and found to be up to the standards. The employer should retain these certificates and be responsible for arranging that the seaman is re-examined at the suggested intervals.

If a potential seaman is found to be unfit it is important that the company be immediately informed and the problem discussed with the candidate. He must be told of the reason for his failure and in particular whether the cause is remediable.

An appeal procedure is available under the Merchant Shipping (Medical Examination) Regulations 1983.

First-Aid Instruction and Training

All crews of stand-by vessels should be instructed in first aid and at least 50% of every crew should have a current first-aid certificate. This should be renewed at intervals not greater than 3 years. The certificates issued by the St. John Ambulance Brigade or British Red Cross Society or other national association are acceptable, but absolute competence and proficiency in cardiopulmonary resuscitation is essential. It is not sufficient that crew members should be instructed solely to obtain a certificate. In addition they should be given special tuition in:

1. The techniques of lifting patients from the water
2. The problems of immersion, considering both drowning and hypothermia
3. Handling of oxygen equipment and stretchers
4. Dealing with oil contamination
5. Triage
6. Transfer of patients to helicopter
7. Seasickness

These medical procedures may have to be performed under conditions of extreme difficulty in wet, cold, dark and pitching vessels, while initial first aid may well have to be carried out on a small, fast rescue boat. It cannot be mentioned too often in the training of crews that immersion victims require the restoration of their ventilation and circulation and the reduction of heat loss. They may be suffering from hypothermia or partial drowning, but with varying degrees of each condition. No attempt need be made to distinguish between these two conditions in the early stage of a rescue. The importance of speedy and persistent resuscitation should be stressed and also it should be made clear that 60% of near-drowners are likely to vomit during the course of resuscitation and that resuscitation should continue until re-warming has occurred. It should be taught that expired air (mouth-to-mouth) remains the best method of ventilation, but can be very difficult in a rigid inflatable in rough weather. The possible need for oxygen after partial drowning should be brought to the crew's attention. The most suitable resuscitator for use on board these vessels is one which is manually operated, time-cycled and can provide 100% oxygen supply of at least 100/l min flow rate. Lifting people who have been in the water for prolonged periods requires extra care, as it is preferable to lift them from the water in a position as nearly horizontal as possible. For this a rigid ladder placed under the casualty may be particularly helpful. The transfer of patients from the sea into rigid inflatables may prove easier by virtue of their low freeboard than onto a stand-by vessel.

Members of the crew need to be specially trained in sorting out casualties (triage), understanding about keeping records of casualties and the recording of details of treatment, possibly by the use of tie-on labels as advocated by the Royal National Life-Boat Institution. The crew should be taught that hypothermic victims should be re-warmed in a bath, no hotter than the hand can bear (41°C), and if necessary their clothes can be cut off while they are in the bath. The baths should allow access from three sides. If baths are not available the patients should be wrapped in blankets and allowed to re-warm spontaneously. This latter method would generally be suitable for casualties who have been in the sea for less than 15 min. Showers are not suitable for re-warming hypothermic casualties.

First-aid training should be conducted by doctors or other persons who are fully conversant with both the offshore and shipping industries, while they also need to know the conditions likely to prevail in a particular area where various stand-by vessels may be serving. The crews of stand-by vessels are keen to learn first aid and other emergency procedures. The problem is that, hopefully, they will get very little practice in dealing with casualties and, therefore, however deep their theoretical knowledge, in practice they have little opportunity to gain experience. It is important that first-aid techniques are practised while crews are at sea, both on board the stand-by vessel and in small, fast rescue boats.

The owner of a stand-by vessel may well use one or more retained company doctors to advise him on the medical aspects of his operations. This adviser should also examine the crew and make arrangements for their first-aid instruction. Employment medical advisers may be prepared to advise on certain problems, but a retained company doctor will probably be more helpful, as he can get to know the members of the crew and undertake most of their instruction himself. Retained doctors may also be able to provide 24 h per day cover for medical advice while the vessels are at sea.

Medical Equipment for Stand-by Vessels

The medical equipment for stand-by vessels is specified in Scale V (or III or IV depending on voyage) of the Merchant Shipping (Medical Scales) Regulation 1974 Statutory Instruction 1193, modified in 1975 to 1581 and 1980 by Statutory Instrument No. 407. Supplementary medical equipment is also necessary:

1. Manual resuscitation apparatus with an adequate supply of oxygen
2. Manual suction apparatus with endotracheal catheters and laryngoscope
3. Laerdal Face Masks and Guerdel airways
4. Intravenous infusion sets with intravenous cannulae; intravenous infusion fluids, e.g. Haemaccel and dextrose saline
5. Stretchers, suitable for transporting patients within the vessel or to another vessel or helicopter
6. Blankets, towels and hot water bottles
7. Hygienic skin and facial cleanser
8. Common and inflatable splints
9. Bandages and dressings as specified in Scale 5, repeated for every 25 survivors or part thereof
10. Urine bottles and bedpans
11. Survival or anti-hypothermia blankets or bags suitably constructed of heat-reflectant and heat-retaining material
12. Parolein eye drops

While individual doctors may feel that they prefer certain brands of medicines, tablets or injections, the Statutory Instruments do provide for a very adequate supply of medical equipment, and it is much easier for companies to comply with statutory regulations applying to all vessels rather than to try and stock for the whims of any particular doctor who may well not be involved in an emergency when it does occur.

The type of fluid used for intravenous replacement is not of particular importance, but the authors have a personal preference for Haemaccel because of its long shelf life and comparative cheapness. It is also considered that the number of bottles prescribed in the regulations is inadequate. It is important that the type of stretcher used can be raised and lowered horizontally (without tilting) as patients may have to be lifted from the decks of stand-by vessels to helicopters, transferred by crane to platforms, or transshipped to lifeboats or other vessels. It is also essential that the stretcher should be manoeuvrable round the sharp bends and angles that occur in stand-by vessels. However, the most important factor about stretchers is that the crew should be accustomed to putting patients into them, and be practised in their use. Patients on ships frequently dislike being on stretchers (preferring if possible to be walking wounded), and it is necessary for the bearers to be competent, kind, gentle and reassuring to their casualties. The medical supplies on stand-by vessels should be regularly reviewed, and drugs should be dated, so that they can be discarded at their expiry date.

Supply Vessels

The same medical standards should be applied to the crew of these vessels as those of stand-by vessels, while a retained company doctor will again be useful. Both supply and stand-by vessels have comparatively small crews of possibly 7–12 people with more on the larger stand-by vessels. It is, therefore, apparent that any unfit member of the crew imposes a serious strain on the remaining members. It is just as important to see that all crew members of supply and stand-by vessels are as fit as those who work on the installations. It is also necessary to remember that when in the course of its duties a supply boat returns to harbour with a sick or injured crew member it is important that he should be dealt with as soon as possible. The supply boat is probably only in the harbour for a short time and either the crew member must be treated and made fit enough to return to work in an often hostile environment or he must be replaced. Figures issued by the Department of Energy show that fatalities and accidents are certainly not uncommon on attendance vessels. Severe accidents are not unusual on board supply vessels and they usually occur in the course of moving heavy loads. While making sure that the crews of such vessels are fit is all important, work accidents cannot be entirely avoided, particularly when bad weather and cranes are involved.

Bibliography

British Medical Journal (1978) Preventing immersion hypothermia. (Editorial) Br Med J II: 1662–1663
Department of Energy, Offshore Technology Paper No. 9: Report and draft guidance notes on the use and effectiveness of stand-by vessels (rescue ships) in offshore operations. November 1981
Harries MG (1979) Mechanical aids to ventilation for use in the field. Br Med J II: 426–428
Hayward JS, Lisson PA, Collis ML, Eckerson JD (1978) Survival suits for accidental immersion in cold water: design concepts and their thermal protection performance. University of Victoria, Canada
Health and Safety Executive (1978) Training of offshore sick-bay attendants (rig medics). HMSO, London (H & S Exec Guidance Note MS16)
Health & Safety Executive (1980) Offshore construction, health, safety and welfare guidelines. HMSO, London (HS (G) 12)
Leese WL, Norman JN (1979) Helicopter passenger survival suit standards in the U.K. offshore oil industry. Aviat Space Environ 2:110–114
Medical Research Council (1976) Survival at sea. Medical Research Council, London.
UKOOA-IAUMED (1984) Survival after helicopter ditching. Report of a workshop held at the Royal College of Physicians, London 15–16 December 1983

Chapter 6

Some Special Problems

R.A.F. Cox and J.N. Norman

Unlike some industries, such as coal mining, some types of chemical manufacturing cotton spinning and rubber processing, which produce the classic diseases of occupation, there are no specific occupational diseases associated with the offshore industry at present. However there are a number of conditions which seem to be particularly common or are related to particular aspects of the industry, and which therefore qualify for special consideration in any account of this subject.

Hydrogen Sulphide

Hydrogen sulphide occurs in so called 'sour gas' in varying concentrations, but in certain parts of the North Sea, the concentration is about 500 parts per million (ppm). It only becomes a problem if it is allowed to escape, when it can be rapidly fatal. Asphyxia occurs at concentrations above 10 ppm and sudden collapse at 600 ppm. It is detectable by the human nose in concentrations of 0.3 ppm. In normal gas production there is normally no leakage of this gas, though at sour gas processing plants a slight smell of hydrogen sulphide is usually detectable. Continuous monitoring for hydrogen sulphide is necessary, with an automatic warning system which activates when the concentration rises above 5 ppm.

During exploration or development drilling in known natural gas reserves, hydrogen sulphide may be inadvertently encountered and uncontrolled release of this material is more likely to occur. In these circumstances, all the workers on a rig may need to wear respirators and they must be medically fit to do so. The theoretical risk of hydrogen sulphide entering the respiratory tract through a perforated tympanic membrane (Poda 1966) is no longer considered significant and potentially exposed workers do not need to be specially examined to ensure that their tympanic membranes are intact.

Hydrogen sulphide is an acute poison which, in concentrations of 600 ppm, may cause sudden asphyxia with collapse, followed by coma and rapidly fatal consequences. At lower concentrations, the eyes become irritated and there is blurring of vision with lachrymation, photophobia and keratitis. As mentioned earlier, the characteristic smell of hydrogen sulphide is detectable in very small concentrations, as low as 0.3 ppm. As the concentration increases, the odour becomes sweeter and more penetrating up to a concentration of 20–30 ppm, but over this concentration olfactory fatigue sets in and the gas may be undetectable. There are no known chronic effects from repeated or continuous inhalation of hydrogen sulphide in low concentrations.

It has recently been pointed out that hydrogen sulphide can be generated in the stagnant water which accumulates in oil storage reservoirs and oil water separators, and also in the legs of offshore platforms and semisubmersibles where there is stagnant seawater. The hydrogen sulphide in these sites is produced by the action of sulphate-reducing bacteria, from the sulphates present in seawater. In stagnant conditions, the aerobic bacteria which are normally present are no longer able to grow, but sulphate-reducing bacteria which metabolise sulphate instead of oxygen can survive, producing hydrogen sulphide and other products. The atmosphere directly above the stagnant water will contain hydrogen sulphide at dangerous levels, and great care must be taken when such areas are entered or opened.

Respirators must be worn in concentrations of 10 ppm.

Radioactivity

Naturally occurring radioisotopes are found in oil and gas reservoirs and in the formation water which they contain. As a result of the production techniques used and, in particular, because of breakthrough of injected seawater into the reservoirs, some of the isotopes may be precipitated and deposited within pipework, valves and pumps. The precipitated scale normally has a low specific activity of less than 74 Bq/g and, even when the equipment is dismantled for maintenance, the dose levels rarely exceed 7.5 μSv/h (7.5×10^{-6} Sieverts/hour). This presents no problem while the system remains closed but, during certain procedures, potential exposure may be sufficient to fall within the compass of the Ionising Radiations Regulations 1985. This is particularly likely during well workovers, when production tubing is pulled from the well, when pipes, pumps or valves are removed, when wells are entered for inspection or cleaning and when the radioactive scale has been removed and requires disposal. Should this be the case, some workers may need to be medically examined by a doctor appointed under the Ionising Radiations Regulations.

At the time of the Chernobyl disaster some installations in Northern waters also experienced a slight rise in radioactivity in the deposits of dust on the air conditioning intake filters. No health hazard was posed.

Methane

Methane is the principal constituent of natural gas, in which its concentration is approximately 85%. It is non-toxic, but it will, of course, produce anoxia if its concentration rises sufficiently high to reduce the partial pressure of oxygen below 150 mmHg. Treatment of anyone overcome by methane is artificial respiration and the administration of oxygen. Methane can produce an explosive mixture with air, and there is a high risk of fire.

Methanol

Methanol is used in gas production to prevent the formation of hydrates in the system, as they could block the pipelines by forming frozen condensates when they mix with water. For practical purposes, methanol is only toxic if ingested. It is known that methanol can be inhaled above its theoretical limit value of 200 ppm without causing illness or discomfort. It cannot be inhaled in sufficiently high quantities to be a toxic hazard via the respiratory route and it is not, in normal usage, absorbed through the skin. Therefore in the offshore situation the toxic effects of methanol are unlikely to be encountered, and those people handling it can be reassured that they are not exposed to any risk in spite of the fact that methanol, when ingested, is highly toxic.

Ethylene Glycol

This is used to absorb water during gas production and like methanol is only toxic, in practice, when ingested. Although the mean lethal dose for an adult is in the region of 100 ml, ethylene glycol is never likely to be ingested in the course of its normal use in gas production processes. It has a low vapour pressure and so does not reach high atmospheric levels. There is no significant absorption through the skin.

Obesity

One rarely hears complaints about the quantity of food offshore, even though there are sometimes complaints about the quality. A large meal may be served every 6 h around the clock, and there are snacks available at all times. Some people expend a considerable number of calories in the course of their work, but many of the workers on a rig have relatively sedentary occupations and excessive weight gain can be a severe problem.

Apart from all the well-recognised dangers of obesity, the obese offshore worker may have difficulty in climbing the large number of stairs, negotiating narrow companionways or even getting comfortable in a 6 × 3-ft bunk. Perhaps, more importantly, he can be a liability in an emergency, for example in a rig evacuation, or if he is the victim of an accident he can be a considerable problem to the stretcher bearers.

In an attempt to reduce the incidence of obesity its dangers must be emphasised and there should be a choice of a low-calorie meal on every menu with its calorific value clearly marked.

Dust

Dust of any sort is not a common problem offshore, but there are a few activities which may create considerable dust. Among these is sandblasting, and the inhalation of dust from this process can cause silicosis. Workers should therefore keep clear of sandblasting operations, and those engaged in the work must wear totally enclosing helmets with a remote supply of air.

Drilling Mud

The other area where dust can be a problem is the mud room, where the dry constituents of the drilling mud are compounded. Any danger here depends entirely upon the nature of the chemicals being handled but, in many cases, precautions will certainly be needed though unfortunately they are often not observed. At the present time the potential exposure of workers to harmful levels of toxic materials in the mud rooms of exploration drilling rigs is a cause of considerable concern. More information about the precise chemical constitution of most constituents of drilling mud is required but some known commonly used substances are:

1. Bentonite, which is a clay derived from volcanic ash and consisting mostly of hydrous aluminium silicates with iron, magnesium, sodium and calcium
2. Barytes, which is barium sulphate
3. Seawater or freshwater
4. Oil is sometimes added to drilling mud
5. Various chemicals including asbestos fibre, various cellulose polymers, carboxy-methylcellulose, lignosulphinates, and diatomaceous earth
6. Various caustic materials

Most mud companies and mud engineers regard the formulation of their compounds as closely guarded proprietary information, which they are reluctant to divulge. There is nevertheless a requirement under the Health and Safety at Work Act to inform workers who are handling these substances of any possible dangers, and it may certainly be necessary to enquire closely into the precise constitution of drilling muds when medical conditions attributable to them occur. Dermatitis, for example, is not uncommon in men who are compounding drilling mud if they do not wear proper protective clothing.

The dust from many drilling muds is an irritant to the eyes and skin. If it gets in the eyes they should be adequately irrigated with water, and contaminated skin should be thoroughly washed. Clothing should be washed before re-use. Chemical goggles and protective clothing must be worn when dry caustic drilling muds are being mixed.

Asbestos was once used regularly in drilling muds. Its use has now been largely discontinued. Other naturally occurring fibres such as attapulgite and palygorskite have been introduced to perform a similar function. From the point of view of potential health hazards, however, these materials should be treated with the same caution as asbestos.

Welding

Welding is a very common offshore operation at all stages, and foreign bodies in the eye from spattering molten metal are common. They are also extremely difficult to remove because, on solidifying, they tend to develop hook-like protuberances which become buried in the cornea. 'Arc eye' also occurs and both of these conditions are easily preventable by wearing suitable protective goggles. Metal fume fever, caused by the exposure of welders to the fumes of the process, which consist of the oxides of the metals being welded and the oxides of nitrogen, may also occur if the welding is being conducted with inadequate ventilation or respiratory protection. Metal fume fever occurs most commonly when zinc, copper, magnesium or their alloys are heated but other metals can also produce the syndrome. It is a self-limiting condition, characterised by fever, rigors, nausea, headache and pains in the limbs.

Noise and Vibration

High noise levels may cause considerable distress, and prevent sleep in the workers on offshore platforms to the extent that some may even require hypnotics or sedatives to prevent insomnia. Apart from causing stress, and perhaps hearing loss, constant high noise levels may interfere with speech and normal conversation and so be a cause of mistakes and accidents.

Although excessively high noise levels may occur in compressor houses and pump rooms, where the wearing of ear defenders must be obligatory, the lower, but still relatively high, noise levels in accommodation areas can be more of a problem. Here, the background noise may produce stress in some individuals and can interfere with normal conversation. The major sources of noise are generators, pumps, compressors and ventilation systems.

In normal, onshore work sites, noise can be calculated to fall off at the rate of about 6 dB each time the distance from the source is doubled. In the offshore situation, this approximate rule does not apply because of the confined and enclosed space, the reflection of sound waves from other structures and the transmission of sound through the framework of the structure itself.

Noise levels offshore must be kept to acceptable levels for the following reasons: (a) to reduce the risk of permanent hearing damage; (b) to prevent interference with essential communication systems; (c) to allow normal voice communication, especially in emergencies; (d) to allow normal sleep and relaxation in recreation and sleeping areas; (e) to ensure that warning signals are audible.

At the present time, noise levels on offshore installations are covered by the Survey Rigs Construction Regulations 1974 and the Offshore Installations (Occupational Health and Safety Welfare Regulations) 1976. In spite of these regulations, surveys on noise levels on offshore platforms have shown ranges considerably in excess of the acceptable limits for shore-based structures.

Recommended noise limits for offshore installations are listed in Table 6.1, and new structures should be designed to meet these recommendations. The relevant section on noise and vibration control from the HMSO publication Offshore Installations: Guidance on Design and Construction is included as Appendix 10.

The nuisance value of noise, and the noise level which is likely to cause complaints, is related more to the relative noise level over the background noise level than it is to its absolute value. In this respect, therefore, the offshore situation is unique because the background value, at least in calm conditions, is very low indeed. Living quarters should be designed so that the noise in living quarters does not exceed 45–50 dB, though with allowances that this level can be exceeded by 5 dB for 25% of the time, 10 dB for 6% of the time and 15 dB for 1.5% of the time to allow for occasional unavoidable excess noise.

Table 6.1. Recommended noise limits on offshore installations

Area	Noise limit (dBA)
General working areas (outside)	88
General working areas (inside) e.g. stores and workshops	70
Kitchens, toilets, laundries, etc.	60
Offices, mess rooms, control rooms	55
Recreation areas	50
Quiet rooms, e.g. radio rooms, conference rooms, sleeping areas, sick bays	45

In general, noisy equipment should be located as far as possible from accommodation and other quiet areas, and so positioned that noise is conducted away from these areas. Quieter machinery areas should be positioned between noisy areas and quiet ones to act as a noise buffer.

Within accommodation areas, quiet rooms such as sick bays and recreation rooms should be separated as far as possible from noisy areas such as kitchens, mess rooms and air-conditioning plants. Living areas may need to be vibration-isolated from the rest of the rig. Specifications for potentially noisy equipment must include proper and adequate noise insulation to keep the noise down to acceptable levels. The cost of modifying a noisy offshore installation to comply with currently accepted noise levels will be very high, and it is imperative to incorporate noise limitation features into the design at the drawing board stage.

Even with the most careful attention to noise control features in the original design, the actual noise levels will not be known until the rig is functioning and it may then be found that, in some areas, noise levels are unacceptably high owing to many factors, including the interaction of different sources and transmission through the structure. To allow for this, plenty of space should be allowed around potential noise sources to permit the installation of noise insulation at a later date.

Where noise levels are unacceptably high and cannot be reduced, ear protection should be mandatory, and such protectors should be provided at the entrance to any noisy areas with clearly written and prominent instructions offering the wearing of such protection.

Trauma

During the exploration and construction phases of offshore oil production, the nature of the work is akin to heavy engineering and construction onshore, and it is therefore not surprising that the type of injuries seen are similar to those in the same industries onshore. The difference is the remoteness of the location in which they occur.

In the drilling phase, heavy, and at times fast-moving machinery is used. Hand and

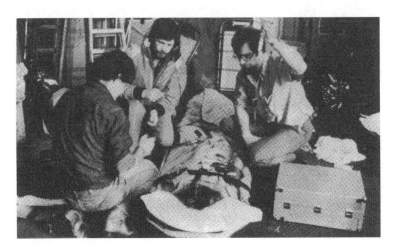

Fig. 6.1. Medics preparing a casualty for transport ashore.

head injuries are common. Heavy loads have to be craned about, including being unloaded from the decks of heaving supply boats. Crushing injuries or trauma from falling objects occur frequently. Decks and stairways can become slippery from grease, oil, drilling mud or ice, and falls occur regularly. When the fall is from one deck to another, the resulting injuries can be very severe if not fatal. In bad weather, which is common, injuries tend to be more frequent, and in all cases the remoteness of the location and the difficulties of transportation introduce serious complications even in the management of relatively minor injuries.

The question of the offshore medics is dealt with elsewhere in this book, and in cases of acute trauma, the patient's survival may depend upon them. Until the arrival of the nearest medic, the victim will depend upon receiving competent first-aid treatment from his colleagues, and it should be general policy to have as many people as possible offshore trained in first aid and holding up-to-date certificates. The role of the first aiders and medics in these cases is to prevent further deterioration in the patient's condition, and to deliver him to the hospital onshore in the best possible state.

Shocked patients travel badly, and the medic must ensure that the patient's condition has been stabilised by arresting bleeding, dressing or splinting wounds as necessary, administering analgesics and intravenous fluids and giving oxygen and artificial respiration as appropriate (Fig. 6.1).

It may be expected that burns would be common in the handling of natural gas and oil, but in fact, the burns cases which have occurred have very rarely been caused by ignition of these products. They have almost all been caused by the careless use of welding torches or the accidental ignition of parts of the living quarters. All cases of burns of 15% or more of the body surface should have an adequate analgesic and an intravenous infusion of a plasma expander set up before commencing the journey ashore.

Scabies and Other Infestations

Scabies is uncommon among the permanent staff of production platforms, but it is endemic among the itinerant employees on exploration drilling rigs and work barges. It is usually contracted ashore, through sexual contact, but can then spread to other members of the crew through the unhygienic habit of 'hot bedding'. This is the use of the same bed by two crew members on opposite shifts — the one frequently getting in as soon as the other one has got out. Although this practice is officially discouraged, it still occurs during periods of intensive manning when the workers may be living in crowded and unhygienic temporary accommodation.

When scabies is diagnosed, it is necessary to inspect any other crew members with rashes of any sort and to disinfect the cabins used by any affected persons. All bedding and clothing should be laundered in the usual way, and mattresses and beds disinfected with liberal quantities of gammabenzene hexachloride. Gammabenzene hexachloride is also the treatment of choice for affected persons and any unaffected persons who have shared a room with an infected colleague (T. Robinson, personal communication).

Pediculosis, usually of the pubic variety, may again occur after a trip ashore. It is less contagious than scabies except among homosexuals, and treatment of the affected person alone is usually sufficient.

Tropical and Other Endemic Diseases in Immigrants

Immigrant labour, usually from Spain, the Middle East, Pakistan, or South America, is common on exploration rigs and work barges. These men are supposed to be medically examined before they leave their home countries, but there is little, if any, check on the quality of the examinations they receive and almost never any documentary clinical evidence. As the employing companies recruit these people in their home countries, there is a natural reluctance to repatriate any who are found to be unfit on arrival at their point of embarkation for the North Sea. Nevertheless, if adequate documentary clinical evidence of their medical examinations cannot be produced before they go offshore, they should be re-examined and, if found unfit, they should be sent back to their country of origin.

Diseases now rare in Europe still tend to be common in many Third World countries, including tuberculosis, poliomyelitis, syphilis, enteric infections and malnutrition. To this list of potential medical disasters in an offshore worker must be added tropical diseases such as schistosomiasis, malaria, amoebiasis and infective hepatitis. Workers recruited in some Third World countries must be regarded from a medical point of view with grave suspicion when it is intended to employ them among a predominantly Western European or North American work force, and in an environment which is totally alien to them. It is not surprising that they do not tolerate the North Sea climate, the isolation, or the separation from their own social culture at all well, and, as a consequence, medical problems both real and imaginary are not uncommon in this group of workers.

It is essential that all workers recruited from countries such as the Middle and Far East for work in the North Sea should be medically examined with extreme care before they leave their country of origin. This examination must include a chest X-ray, a haematology profile, and screening for Australia antigen in addition to a thorough history and physical examination. The physicians hired to perform these examinations should be reviewed and appointed by a medical representative of the employers, whose responsibility it is to ensure that medical standards are maintained.

The examining doctor may encounter many problems in connection with these workers. He must constantly bear in mind the tropical and other diseases already mentioned in considering his differential diagnosis. In addition, he must be aware that, for the reasons discussed above, malingering is common and not easy to recognise, and the whole consultation may be conducted through an interpreter. Finally, he may be faced with a problem of disposal because the patient may not have a visa. The patient may not be ill enough to justify hospital admission, and the immigration authorities may insist that he may only stay onshore if he is admitted to hospital or jail. If there is a possibility that he is infectious, it may be impossible to find accommodation for him in a hotel or lodging house. It is not unknown for the doctor to be stranded with the patient in his examination room with a policeman outside and the company representative having disappeared. Contractors frequently lose all interest in their workers when they cease to work, and cannot understand why the local hospital cannot relieve them of their responsibilities towards any person who is ill. The hospital admitting officer must, quite rightly, satisfy himself that the person qualifies for admission purely on medical grounds, while the immigration authorities are required to keep an illegal immigrant under surveillance. The safest place, from their point of view, is police custody. In fact responsibility for these people rests firmly with the employers, who should ascertain before they leave their home countries (a) that they are medically fit, (b) that they have visas for any country to which they might be evacuated in an emergency, and (c) that arrangements have been made with a local private nursing home where they can be admitted and cared for by the employers' local retained physician.

Psychological Disturbances

In 1970 the North Sea Medical Centre reviewed the reasons for the evacuation of offshore workers, and found that acute psychological disturbance was second only to trauma. With better selection of people, better working conditions and a more experienced pool of offshore workers, it is believed that psychological problems are less common now, but the offshore environment is still a rough and tough world likely to tax the mental equilibrium of any person who is not wholly stable. Conditions on mobile drilling rigs are not very comfortable, there is a lack of privacy, a mixed community of very different people, socially and intellectually, constant noise, and arduous work interspersed with periods of great boredom. These are just the right conditions for producing anxiety and depression in susceptible individuals. Those who usually succumb are intelligent, often professional types such as engineers or geologists, sensitive and introspective. Some may have a fear of flying, especially in helicopters, and the prospect of the weekly helicopter ride may be the last straw.

Overt psychosis is not uncommon, as exemplified by the following three cases:

1. A 25-year-old geologist who, after a period of increasing withdrawal, climbed the derrick and refused to come down until he had spoken to the Chairman of the company.

2. A 23-year-old Israeli who, at the time of the Egypt–Israel war, jumped overboard 'to swim to the help of my countrymen'. After being rescued he then severed one of the fuel lines to the barge's engines when the captain refused to set sail for Israel.

3. A 28-year-old diver who, under the influence of drugs, attacked one of his colleagues with an axe. He was only restrained when he was persuaded to remove his wetsuit and was overpowered when his trousers were round his ankles.

In some cases it is wives who worry about their husbands flying in helicopters, and the practice of insisting that all passengers wear immersion suits tends to raise the anxiety level. Passengers, not unreasonably, imagine that the helicopter flights are much more dangerous than scheduled flights in other aircraft, although this is not borne out by the statistics. In the opinion of the authors, it is debatable whether the possible potential advantages of an immersion suit in a helicopter crash outweigh the disadvantage of raising passenger anxiety.

An acutely disturbed patient on an offshore rig poses a difficult management problem. The patient must be calm, and sedated if necessary, before attempting to bring him ashore. The best sedative is probably haloperidol or chlorpromazine. This is an occasion when, for clinical and medico-legal reasons, the presence of a doctor is essential.

Drugs and Alcohol

Both drugs and alcohol are strictly forbidden offshore, but it must be admitted that they are smuggled out at times, even when the penalty for being caught is instant dismissal.

There is little evidence that hard drugs are a serious problem, though 'pot' is undoubtedly in frequent use, perhaps especially among the divers. A recent random survey for cannabis residue in urine among offshore drilling crews revealed an incidence of 12% (Calder 1986). Analytical techniques for the detection of cannabis are very sensitive, and traces are detectable on hands for 48 h, in urine for 3 days and in blood for 1 week after smoking the resin. There is no doubt that drug abuse in the offshore situation can lead to some very dangerous operational and legal liability situations, and it should not be tolerated under any circumstances. Under the Misuse of Drugs Act it is illegal to permit the smoking of cannabis on one's premises. So, if a company or an OIM is aware that such acts are taking place, they can be held liable and subject to a gaol sentence. Spot checks of baggage and the swabbing of hands are valuable deterrents, and offenders should face instant dismissal. The random detection of drug abusers is, however, a matter for the security and personnel departments, not the medical.

Enforced abstinence from alcohol and the relatively high wages of offshore workers encourages some to drink heavily when they are onshore. Some offshore workers, in Scotland, are reputed to be almost permanently inebriated during their days on leave, and only dry out again when they get back to the rig. Aiken and McCance (1982), following their investigation into alcohol consumption by offshore workers, stated 'many workers must be arriving offshore in a post-alcoholic state unsuited to the demands and dangers of the job'. The offshore industry may have exacerbated the very serious problem of excessive drinking from which Scotland has always suffered.

Itinerant workers on mobile rigs and barges are particularly difficult to help, but permanent employees on fixed installations are more amenable to assistance with their problem. Every company should have a policy to help those of its employees who have a drinking problem. The policy should enable the patient to seek help through the company without prejudice or fear of suffering any financial penalty. The policy should also encompass instructions to supervisors in improving their awareness of the problem, recognising the symptoms, and broaching the subject in a helpful, sympathetic and uncritical manner.

Medical officers acting on behalf of a company in respect of its alcohol policy must acknowledge alcoholism as a disease, must accept employees who may be referred to them with the observance of customary strict medical confidentiality, and must have a pre-prepared route of referral.

Drugs and drink problems are symptoms of the social malaise which afflicts our society at this time, but the standards to which a small offshore community must adhere do not permit any tolerance of the destructive and disruptive influence of these substances.

Partial Drowning and its Treatment

When an offshore worker falls from an installation into the North Sea the main problem is usually to find him. The seas in the northern North Sea have waves greater that 1 m in height for more than 90% of the time, and recovery of a person falling into the sea may take anything up to $1\frac{1}{2}$ h even though his entry into the water has been observed. Most commonly, such accidents result in loss of the subject. If he is recovered from the water, however, he may be suffering from drowning, from hypothermia, from the traumatic effects of a fall from a height of around 150 ft, or from a combination of these effects, so the initial problem may be one of diagnosis.

Helicopter ditching also involves the danger of drowning, or partial drowning, even though an adequate life jacket is worn together with a helicopter passenger survival suit. It was held until recently that the main danger under these circumstances was that of hypothermia, but the trachea is so close to the surface of the sea that with high wind speeds and consequent spray it is not easy to avoid aspiration of sea water. This may occur early in immersion, and would thus be likely to play an increasing part in the pathological picture as time passes.

The management of the subject removed from the water and found to be unconscious follows the standard line of resuscitation, bearing in mind the possibility of traumatic injury and of hypothermia. Drowning, by definition, is death from acute asphyxia while submerged, whether or not fluid has entered the lungs. The term 'partial drowning' is applied to those individuals who survive immersion.

The emergency care of the partial drowning victim should be airway clearance and mouth-to-mouth resuscitation or mouth-to-nose ventilation. Artificial ventilation should always be started as soon as possible — even before the victim is removed from the water. Following the institution of standard artificial ventilation the patient should, if pulseless, receive external cardiac massage. It has recently been suggested that the period in which resuscitation may be effective could be extended if drowning had taken place in very cold water. This emphasises the need for prolonged resuscitative attempts which should, if possible, be continued until death is pronounced by a doctor.

Drowning victims often swallow large volumes of water, and their stomachs usually become distended. This impairs ventilation and circulation and should be alleviated as soon as possible. If water has been inhaled into the lungs, attempts at postural drainage waste valuable time and are of little value.

Immediate First Aid

Respiration

The initial check and clearance of any airway obstruction should be followed by mouth-to-mouth respiration — the ventilation rate should be approximately 12–14 breaths per minute, with increased rates in the very young.

Circulation

If no pulse is detected, external cardiac massage should be performed at a rate of 60–80 strokes per minute. In combined cardiopulmonary resuscitation the adult rates should be: with one operator, 2 breaths per 15 compressions of the sternum; with two operators, 1 breath per 6 compressions of the sternum.

Secondary Drowning

An attempt should always be made to move the patient to hospital once immediate resuscitation measures have been instigated, as it may be necessary to implement more intensive therapy, particularly if secondary drowning occurs.

Following a successful resuscitation, it is important to consider the possibility of secondary drowning. Much used to be made of the distinction between freshwater drowning and seawater drowning, from the differences which absorption of fresh or saltwater across the respiratory tract made in the electrolyte composition of the blood. It is now felt that this is of little importance and, in any event, the larynx may go into spasm as soon as contact is made with cold water, so that the amount of water in the lungs may not in fact be great. If a considerable amount of water has entered the lungs, whether it is salt or fresh, the main secondary phenomenon which is likely to occur is that of secondary drowning. The victim often appears quite well shortly after resuscitation and the dangers of secondary drowning are not widely appreciated. The condition is due to the possible aspiration of vomit, mud, sand, diatoms and aquatic vegetation in addition to water, causing an outpouring of colloid fluid from the irritated pulmonary epithelium and interference with the surfactant mechanism. The resultant picture resembles that of aspiration of vomit during anaesthesia (Mendelson's syndrome).

Secondary drowning can occur from 15 min to 4 days after the near-drowning incident, and survival depends upon the rapid institution of active measures. It is thus very important when a patient has been successfully resuscitated in a remote place that he be sent immediately to hospital, since the development of this condition may require urgent measures and a prolonged period of artificial ventilation. It has recently been suggested that the secondary drowning phenomenon could be avoided if the patient were given an immediate dose of steroids (Oliver et al. 1978). It has also been shown that the effect of steroids in pharmacological dosage in the management of the refractory shock is time-related (Smith and Norman 1979). Since time and distance is a major problem in offshore medicine, an intravenous dose of 2 g methylprednisolone together with 500 mg ampicillin intramuscularly may be considered to be a useful prophylactic against secondary drowning, following a successful resuscitation offshore. It would seem reasonable to recommend such treatment before the patient is transported to a shore-based hospital. Secondary drowning emphasises the importance of rapid transfer of the partially drowned patient to hospital after successful resuscitation, even though there are no abnormal signs or symptoms. The use of steroids in drowning, as in other acute conditions, has been widely debated, but only small doses have been used in the past and this may account for the apparent lack of response noted. The value of pharmacological doses of methylprednisolone in acute situations has steadily gained clinical acceptance, and the importance of its early administration has been noted. In its worst form, secondary drowning may require a prolonged period of artificial ventilation.

Hypothermia

The deep body temperature of man is a dynamic balance, and results from metabolic heat production and those thermal losses to the environment sustained by conduction, convection and radiation. Despite the wide variation in heat production caused by different human activities, and the extensive range of environmental conditions within which man has chosen to live or work, the diurnal variation of body temperature is of the order of 1°C. Such precision of internal temperature regulation is necessary for the optimum function of the human body, since this is basically a matter of a rather complex variety of temperature-sensitive enzymes.

Physiologically, body temperature is maintained within its narrow range by varying the state of activity voluntarily or involuntarily in the form of exercise or shivering, respectively, and also by changing the state of surface insulation by varying the degree of blood flow through the subcutaneous tissues. In addition to purely physiological mechanisms, man has used his intelligence to allow him to penetrate to the coldest areas of the earth with safety by taking his microenvironment with him by the use of clothing, artificial heating and housing. When all the voluntary and involuntary physiological and intellectual mechanisms fail and the body temperature falls, a state of hypothermia is said to have been achieved when the body temperature falls to 35°C or below.

The clinical manifestations of early hypothermia are sometimes not easy to determine and are usually mental in origin. The subject may become abnormally aggressive and argumentative, or alternatively he may become unusually withdrawn and apathetic. The important factor is that of change in personality and this proceeds, as the temperature falls, through a period of mental confusion to unconsciousness, which may take place anywhere below 32°C. The question of loss of judgement or competence with modest degrees of body cooling has been argued over for many years in relation to hill walkers, and has received much attention recently with regard to the aetiology of accidents on offshore structures. So far, however, there has been no convincing demonstration of loss of cognitive function with moderate hypothermia, other than the possible distracting effect of the associated discomfort. This is a matter, however, which needs some urgent definition, for offshore workers are now frequently called upon to operate equipment which requires considerable skill in very cold conditions. In addition to the question of judgement and competence, there are specialised offshore situations, such as a diving bell on the seabed bereft of power, where survival may depend upon the performance of a manoeuvre, such as opening a gas bottle or adjusting the oxygen tension in the atmosphere. Under these conditions, the duration of survival may be related more to the deterioration of intellectual function than to cardiac arrest at a temperature which may be as much as 10°C lower.

Shivering normally occurs during the early stages of hypothermia, and this may require an increase in tissue oxygen supply of as much as 300% over basal levels. There is thus a considerable demand placed upon the heart early in the application of cold stress, and it seems possible that people with an already damaged myocardium could be at risk from the cold even before the body temperature begins to fall. When the temperature falls, the nerve conduction rate is reduced and the heart rate falls in sympathy with temperature. As long as shivering persists, however, there is considerable demand for oxygen by the muscles, which may remain until the body temperature approaches 30°C. Thus, in the case of accidental hypothermia, as opposed to deliberately induced hypothermia in the operating theatre where muscle relaxation is used, the oxygen consumption may be as great at 30°C as at normothermia. The cardiac output will thus be similar to the output at normothermia also, and since cold will have depressed the rate, the stroke volume will have increased. It is probably for reasons such as these that the heart is so vulnerable in hypothermia, and death usually occurs from asystole or ventricular fibrillation at a temperature somewhere below 33°C. The actual point of arrest may, of course, be at a very much lower temperature.

It is not easy to find an acceptable means of monitoring the body temperature in people at work or recreation in a cold environment. Mouth temperature is most unreliable in a cold climate since it is so much affected by the saliva which reflects the temperature of the glands close to the surface of an exposed area. Expired air temperature is lower than core temperature, but bears a constant relationship to core temperature in the steady state. This relationship is not constant when the ventilation rate changes, however, and this is implied in field work. Urine temperature has been used with some success and tympanic temperature is rather uncomfortable and not acceptable in underwater workers in view of the ear complaints which divers can acquire. Rectal temperature is currently the only reliable means of monitoring deep body temperature in this field, but it tends to be unacceptable unless for well-founded experimental purposes.

These problems of measurement have meant that much reliance is placed upon a worker's personal, subjective assessment of his thermal status. This assessment is based upon cutaneous sensation and the presence or absence of shivering. It has been pointed out recently that a goodly proportion of fit young subjects do not shiver in response to severe cold stress, and it has been known for many years that the sensory end-organs of the trunk appear to be more attuned to the detection of rapid change of environmental temperature than to the registration of its absolute value. It has also been pointed out that those who shiver violently often complain most of serious discomfort in the cold, but tend to maintain their body temperature longer than those who do not shiver. It thus seems clear that the human may not always be a reliable witness of his state of thermal balance, and may even be in a state of hypothermia without realising it. This is particularly true if the rate of change of temperature is slow, and could be important in the aetiology of accidents in working situations where a degree of judgement is needed. It could also be an important consideration in heliox-breathing divers, since the temperature of the hot water which perfuses their suits is almost entirely related to the divers' subjective sensation of heat or cold.

When a subject walks or is at work in a cold, dry situation, there are several factors which will determine whether he can maintain his body temperature or whether he will gradually cool. Aside from the two important factors of the severity of the climate to which he is actually exposed and the efficiency of the clothing assembly with which he is provided, an important variable will be the level of activity which he can maintain, which is, of course, a measure of his state of physical fitness. The fit man will be able to sustain a high level of physical exertion and maintain his body temperature, while his less fit colleague may not be able to produce sufficient heat to balance his losses and will slowly cool. Physical fitness is thus an important determinant of survival in a cold climate, and it seems possible that the state of nutrition and body composition may also be involved, but this is less certain. Whether motivation plays the important part in survival potential claimed for it by some is not clear. It seems equally possible that the point where a victim of exposure/exhaustion collapses may be determined entirely by his state of fitness, nutrition and body composition together with factors relating to clothing and the environment. If motivation plays a part, however, it ought to be capable of identification and measurement, and thus of value in selection procedures for tasks involving serious degrees of environmental stress.

The cooling power of the environment on man is an important measure, and is fraught with difficulties. Ambient temperature and wind velocity are the two main determinants currently considered in this context, and their combined effect is sometimes expressed in the wind-chill index. This is a most convenient method of indicating the combined effects of wind velocity and temperature, and the wind-chill scale is widely used to give an indication of the order of magnitude of the cooling power of these two parameters. The objection to the application of this scale to man is that it is based on the cooling power of various environmental conditions on non-insulated cans of water, which obviously have no metabolism. It is, therefore, not possible to translate such values to man with any accuracy, since in the case of man, the rate of cooling in response to change of environment varies in relation to metabolic rate, clothing worn, variation in physiological insulation and possibly also to the state of acclimatisation. The net result is that the cooling values at the top of the scale tend to be too high, since at the coldest temperatures man has a physiological protection by which he can conserve his heat. The problem of expressing the combined effects of wind velocity and temperature on man in terms of a single factor has thus not yet been solved completely.

Physiological meteorology is nevertheless an important subject, since serious errors have been made in supplying equipment to polar stations when the choice has resulted from considering conventional meteorological data, such as maximum and minimum values of temperature and wind velocity. Considerable resource has been needlessly spent in the past in supplying equipment and living accommodation capable of withstanding, say, −60°C and 70 knots wind velocity, in areas where these values have been known to occur. What was not known was that they may have occurred separately for an almost insignificant length of time and probably never together. Frequency data rather than mean data are thus required if the true climatic picture is to be appreciated. These would indicate, for example, the range of temperature for each period of time and its duration. From the physiological viewpoint, it is much more meaningful to be able to say that a man was exposed to, say, 10°C for 30% of the time and to −20°C for 70% of the time than that he was exposed to −17°C as an average.

Given a knowledge of the activity patterns of a place, then, by the use of frequency data, one can begin to arrive at a concept of the exposure. Similar frequency data are, of course, required for wind velocity, which is certainly the chief cause of discomfort and the main governor of outside work potential in cold regions. It is also a most significant factor in body cooling.

Though both of these analyses are important in themselves, probably the most significant of all are double-frequency analyses of wind velocity and temperature. The frequency with which combinations of low temperature and high wind velocity occur together is important in the assessment of man's actual exposure to cold, and to the provision of suitable clothing, equipment and living accommodation for a given remote station. No less significant, of course, is the observation of the frequency with which: (a) high temperatures accompany low wind velocity; (b) high temperatures accompany high wind velocity; and (c) low temperatures accompany low wind velocity. For a given place, an integrated view of all these parameters makes it possible to build up a picture of the likely exposure of a man to that particular environment.

The clothing assembly worn is of great importance in a hostile climate, and much work is currently being undertaken in the design of new fabrics. Windproof fabric provided the first major advance in this field and this took account of both temperature and wind velocity. The effect of water has received much consideration, but as yet no effective measure of the cooling power of the environment has been developed which takes dampness into account in addition to wind and temperature. Water is a better conductor than air by a factor of 25 and the insulative value of a clothing assembly is largely determined by the amount of still air which it can trap in its interstices. The thorough wetting of a clothing assembly and the replacement of air by water will have the effect of reducing its insulative value to 10% of its control value. Modern technology has produced a fabric known as Goretex, which claims to be waterproof and windproof and yet to allow the evaporation of sweat from within to outside. Such developments will undoubtedly eventually allow man to work with comfort and safety within any given range of environmental variables.

Treatment

Hypothermia sometimes results in complex disturbances of the body's economy and it is probably managed with greatest success when the patient has been admitted to the intensive care unit of a well-found hospital with adequate laboratory back-up. Even under these circumstances, however, there is still considerable disagreement about the best method of managing the condition. However, the hospital care of hypothermia will not be discussed at this time because the problem which requires to be addressed is the management of hypothermia when it occurs in a remote work site or when the facilities available for management are those of an offshore sick bay. From what has been said previously, it is clear that the most vulnerable organ when the body temperature is reduced to hypothermic levels is the heart, which is in a state of irritability and under considerable stress. It is particularly liable to develop ventricular fibrillation at any time during the cooling or the re-warming phases. Cardiac arrest is likely to supervene only when the temperature falls to relatively low levels, provided always that the heart was in an undamaged state before the body temperature was lowered. A further problem is the extreme difficulty of defibrillation of the hypothermic heart. All this implies a need to provide treatment as soon as possible. This means treatment offshore or as soon after rescue as is practical in a remote work site. It has to be remembered that the responsible medical officer may be based at a considerable distance from the site of the hypothermic accident and treatment may have to be undertaken by a rig medic or even on occasions by laymen. This in turn implies a need for training in re-warming techniques, the establishment of a clear policy and the presence of good communications between the offshore and onshore sites.

It seems clear that much of the controversy which has taken place in the past about the management of hypothermia has been due to a failure to realise that hypothermia is not a single state, but a group of very different clinical entities characterised only by the common factor of a low body temperature. When this fact is accepted treatment becomes easier. It is only necessary to determine the cause of the hypothermia and treat that particular clinical entity within the syndrome. There are at least four entirely different clinical conditions which result in hypothermia and which require different methods of treatment:

Immersion

When the casualty is immersed in cold water the body temperature tends to fall rapidly. This is due to the high thermal conductivity of water which is at least 25 times greater than air. Under these circumstances the body will cool if the temperature of the water is below the thermoneutral point of 32.8°C. This is why hypothermia can still occur following prolonged immersion in tropical waters. In the waters of the North Sea, however, where the temperature is very much colder and may vary between 4° and 12°C, the body will cool very rapidly and reach hypothermic levels before there has been time for any considerable degree of metabolic change or physiological adjustment to take place. This implies that the safest means of treating the condition is to reverse the thermal gradient as rapidly as possible by re-immersion in hot water so that the heart is not left in a vulnerable state for any longer than is necessary. Since the condition will have taken place rapidly there is little risk of complications arising from metabolic or circulatory adjustments due to the hypothermia.

Another factor which needs to be considered at this time is the occurrence of the condition known as post-rescue death and which has been studied most intensively by Golden and Hervey (1981). This is a condition which has been noted most frequently in association with shipwreck. It often occurs in those who have been recovered on board a rescue vessel in a conscious state and apparently relatively unharmed, but some little time later they collapse and die. This condition is much more commonly associated with the immersion incident than with any other type of hypothermia. It has been suggested that the cause is associated with the vulnerability of the cooled heart. The effort of rescue usually requires the subject to climb up some form of scrambling net or to use considerable physical force to achieve the deck of the rescue vessel. In addition, extraction of the casualty from the water results in the removal of the hydrostatic pressure caused by the water, and this may in turn reduce the venous return. The collapse is then said to be due to the combined effects of cold on the function of the heart, physical exertion required by the subject in getting out of the water and removal of the hydrostatic pressure caused by the water. This possibility adds another cogent argument for recommending immediate re-immersion of the casualty in warm water.

Re-immersion is best carried out in a bath which is free on all sides so that the attendants can stand all round. This can be achieved, where accommodation is limited, by the use of an inflatable bath which can be stored in a small space when it is not required. It is important that the body core should be re-warmed preferentially, and for this reason it is recommended that the trunk should be placed in the bath with the arms and legs remaining outside in the first instance, if this is possible.

The recommended water temperature is 42°C, but in practice it will be found that this will cause intense discomfort to the hypothermic skin, and it is probably best to begin with water at around the normal body temperature of 37°C. The water temperature can then gradually be increased towards 42°C, as the casualty becomes more able to accept increased heat. This technique may not be practical if there is a limited supply of hot water when the extreme discomfort may just have to be endured. If hot water is freely available it should also be remembered that it will cool very rapidly, and that it will require constant adjustment. A further point of some practical importance is that it is not really necessary to remove the casualty's clothing before placing him in the bath, and in many ways the added exertion of removing wet clothing may just tip the balance and precipitate ventricular fibrillation. This arrhythmia will be almost impossible to reverse if the temperature is below 30°C, even though the equipment may be available to attempt this procedure. Following re-warming to normal temperature the casualty should be allowed to rest in bed, in a warm room for at least 48 h.

Exposure/Exhaustion

When hypothermia occurs during walking or working in cold air it usually develops very slowly. This is because air is a poor conductor and the subject is continuously increasing his activity, in order to combat the cooling power of the environment. Only when that cooling power becomes greater than the victim's ability to increase his activity does the body slowly cool. This slow process only takes place after all the protective and compensatory mechanisms have been brought into play and there are resultant circulatory and metabolic changes which become more intense as the body cools. The intense vasoconstriction of the periphery which provides for an increase in the insulation of the body core, is associated with a reduction in blood volume. This is because the capacity of the circulatory space is now reduced by the vasoconstriction.

This is reflected by the well-known cold diuresis. If the subject is rapidly re-warmed there is a real possibility of developing hypovolaemic shock since there is likely to be insufficient fluid in the circulatory space to fill it completely when it dilates. This does not matter in hospital where an intravenous line can readily be established, but it may be a factor worthy of consideration in the remote place, and it would suggest that a slower rate of re-warming would be preferable so that circulatory haemodynamics can be given time for re-establishment by means of the addition of the necessary fluid by the alimentary tract, rather than intravenously. The constriction of the circulation, particularly in the limbs, results in tissue hypoxia and consequently anaerobic metabolism of the peripheral tissues. It is often suggested that rapid re-warming may cause a flushing of these acid metabolites into the core of the body before the liver has re-warmed adequately to deal with them, and this may allow them to exert their fibrillating effect on the cold heart. It is for this reason that if rapid re-warming by immersion is chosen, then the arms and the legs are normally left cold until the core organs, and particularly the liver and heart, have been re-warmed. Exposure/exhaustion is in fact such a complex state that it is far from being adequately understood as yet. In addition to the hypothermic component there is a considerable biochemical disturbance which is likely to be associated with the fatigue element of the condition. For these reasons it would be best managed in a remote place by slow re-warming. Every attempt should be made to keep the patient calm and free from excessive exertion. He should be placed in a warm sleeping bag and observed carefully until a normal body temperature has been established, and thereafter as before, given at least 48 h bed rest to allow full recovery to take place.

Hypothermia Occurring in Divers

The hypothermia associated with deep diving is caused by entirely different mechanisms from any other since the respiratory tract becomes increasingly important in heat exchange with depth as the density of the gases increases. Below 50 m depth, when helium is breathed the respiratory tract becomes the most important mechanism of heat exchange owing to the sixfold increase in both specific heat and thermal conductivity of helium over air. The diver is normally kept warm by the use of a suit heated either by electricity or hot water, this supplies heat to the surface of the body to compensate for that lost by the respiratory tract.

It should be noted that respiratory heat gain or loss at atmospheric pressure can never be greater than 10% of metabolic heat production and this relationship does not change with ventilation rate. The respiratory tract is therefore not an important avenue of heat loss at atmospheric pressure. For the same reasons, attempts which have been made to use the respiratory tract as a means of re-warming the hypothermic victim in the field have proved disappointing at atmospheric pressure.

Urban Hypothermia

When hypothermia occurs in cities it is often in the elderly living in underheated housing and in association with disease of the circulatory or nervous system. It may also occur in association with such disease processes as myxoedema or in those who have consumed alcohol or narcotics in excessive quantities. The mechanisms for producing hypothermia and the management of associated disease processes constitute an entirely different clinical situation from the previous three. It is not, however, a condition which is often found offshore and, therefore, its management will not be considered further at this point.

It thus appears that much of the controversy associated with the management of hypothermia is due to a failure in the past to appreciate the considerable differences in the clinical states which result from reduction of the body temperature by different means. It seems likely that management will be just as different for each type of hypothermia.

Bibliography

Aiken GJM, McCance C (1982) Alcohol consumption in offshore oil rig workers. Br J Addict 77: 305–310
Auld CD, Light IM, Norman JN (1979) Accidental hypothermia and rewarming in dogs. Clin Sci 56: 601–606
Calder IM (1986) to be published
Golden FStC, Hervey GR (1981) The after-drop and death after rescue from immersion in cold water. In: Adam EJ (ed) Hypothermia — ashore and afloat. Aberdeen University Press, Aberdeen pp 37–56
Keatinge WR (1969) Survival in cold water. Blackwell, Oxford
Norman JN, Brebner JA (1985) The offshore health handbook. Martin Dunitz, London
Oliver E, Miller JDB, Norman JN (1978) Steroids and secondary drowning. Lancet I: 105–106
Poda GA (1966) Hydrogen sulphide can be handled safely. Arch Environ Health 12: 795–800
Ronk R, White MK (1985) Hydrogen sulfide and the probabilities of inhalation through a tympanic membrane defect. J Occup Med 27: 337–340
Smith JAR, Norman JN (1979) Use of glucocorticoids in refractory shock. Surgery 149: 363–373

Chapter 7

Diving

P.B. James and R.A.F. Cox

Diving Techniques

Diving has been required for almost all of the thousands of wells drilled offshore since the first oilfield development in the Gulf of Mexico in 1948. In the last decade a small number of wells have been drilled in water depths from 300 to 1500 m without the support of conventional divers by using 1-atm vehicles ranging from armoured suits to small submarines. As these devices operate at a pressure very close to atmospheric pressure, no compression and decompression is required. Although they continue to improve there is always likely to be a requirement for divers because they can work in confined spaces and low visibility.

In drilling operations diving is only needed occasionally to correctly position and align the in-water structures which comprise the blowout preventer and riser casing. Diving may be required to maintain this structure during the drilling of a hole and, after completion of the operation, in the recovery of the machinery and casing. The dives are usually of short duration with typical bottom times of between 30 min and 1 h.

In construction diving, divers are more often required in the positioning of structures and to make the many pipeline connections on the seabed under the production platform. A major function is the retrieval of items dropped into the sea.

Once the oilfield is in production there is a constant requirement for inspection and maintenance. Inspection is usually by a diver carrying photographic and ultrasonic equipment. Corrosion rates are high and steel structures require the attachment of anodic protection — large pieces of zinc, which require regular renewal. Cracks may develop in the structure as a result of continuous flexion and may require considerable additional bracing and grouting. In the last few years hyperbaric welding techniques have been successfully used to depths of over 300 m. The following diving techniques need to be considered.

SCUBA Diving

The initials stand for self-contained underwater breathing apparatus, indicating that the diver carries his own gas supply. This type of diving is little used in offshore work because of the very limited duration possible and the difficulty of providing an adequate reserve gas supply to cover emergencies. Good communications are required in commercial diving, and they are difficult to provide in the free-swimming

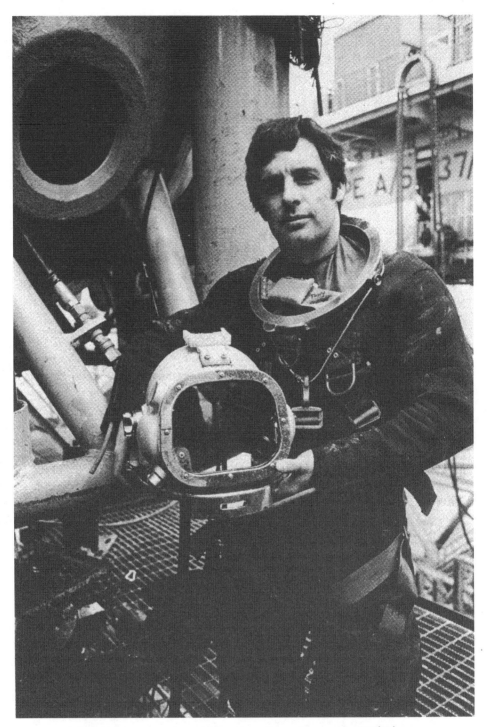

Fig. 7.1. Modern diver wearing a heated suit and carrying an Oceaneering 'rat hat'.

diver. Once a lifeline and communication lines are used it becomes logical to add an air supply hose. The cylinder carried on the diver's back then becomes an emergency supply in the event of a main supply failure. The clothing worn by the diver depends upon the water temperature. In warm water often a coverall may be all that is required. In cooler water a wet suit may be used, but for very cold water constant-volume dry suits are necessary.

Surface-Orientated Surface-Supplied Diving

In this form of diving the diver is provided with an umbilical carrying his breathing gas and communications. Free-flooding hot water suits may also be used, which require a supply of hot water from the surface (Fig. 7.1). The diver is tended from the surface and it is normal for a fully dressed stand-by diver to be on site for emergencies. The old-fashioned 'hard hat' deep-sea gear, invented by John Deane about 1820 and subsequently developed by Augustus Siebe, is now rarely used (Fig. 7.2), but it

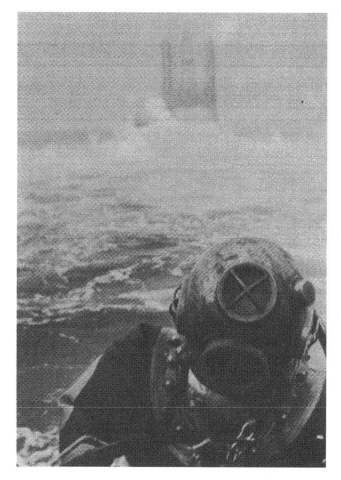

Fig. 7.2. Diver in standard diving gear on 'North Sea Bubble' with drilling rig Constellation in the background.

has the advantage of containing enough gas to allow the diver to breathe for about 15 min in the event of stoppage of the surface supply. It also provides excellent protection in salvage work and harbour clearance, where feeling is more important than seeing. It has now largely been replaced by masks and helmets made of glass-reinforced plastic. A helmet is always to be preferred to a mask in commercial diving, for a mask is too easily dislodged and the diver is then liable to drown.

Surface-orientated diving is limited in the United Kingdom to 50 m (165 ft) and in the United States to 60 m (200 ft). These depths also represent the maximum depths to which compressed air may be used in the respective countries. There can be little doubt that this type of diving is the most dangerous from many standpoints. Diving close to the surface may render the diver's buoyancy difficult to control and this, combined with the action of wave and swell, may also make transfer into and out of the water dangerous. This may be obviated partially by the use of a diving stage or 'wet bell' lowered and raised by a winch. Serious decompression sickness is also more common in this type of diving with compressed air.

Surface-supplied diving is commonly used in conjunction with a chamber to allow the technique of surface decompression to be used. The technique was devised in 1925 to allow a diver to be removed from cold water, recompressed and finally decompressed in a warm chamber. In practice this recompression is a treatment for the gas separated from solution by the omission of the correct decompression stoppages in the original dive.

Submersible Decompression Chambers and Deck Chambers

A diving system consists of a diving bell or personnel transfer capsule and one or more deck chambers attached to a transfer lock. The use of a bell allows the diver to be tended by a colleague, who can often watch him at work. The bell provides a safe refuge containing a respirable gas underwater, and also a means of transfer through the water interface in relative comfort and safety. 'Locking' the bell onto the deck chamber on the surface allows transfer under pressure to be achieved without the divers being decompressed to atmospheric pressure.

The dive may be either a sub-saturation or a saturation exposure. In a sub-saturation or 'bounce' dive, the diver does not equilibrate with the partial pressures of the gases supplied at the bottom depth and is able to decompress relatively quickly back to atmospheric pressure. For example, an exposure of 30 min at 150 m (492 ft) which includes the compression time of about 5 min, requires about 15 h in decompression. A diver saturated or equilibrated at the same depth will require about 3 days in decompression, but this time will be the same regardless of the time spent at depth. Saturation dives last from a few hours to 60 days, but there is a tendency for the duration to be limited to a maximum of about 21 days. It is usual to use an intermediate depth for storage in the living chambers on deck. The divers on a 'bell-run' then have to pressurise the bell close to bottom depth before locking-out. A typical bell-run lasts 7–8 h with the divers in the bell sharing the work. The bell is then lifted and is used by a second pair of divers working on an opposite shift. This ensures the maximum utilisation of both divers and equipment. The use of a free-flooding hot water suit and gas heating ensures that the diver can remain comfortable for long periods, even in very cold water. Provided the gas mixtures supplied are correct and mechanical failures do not occur, saturation diving is the safest method of diving for the number of hours spent in the water (Figs. 7.3–7.6).

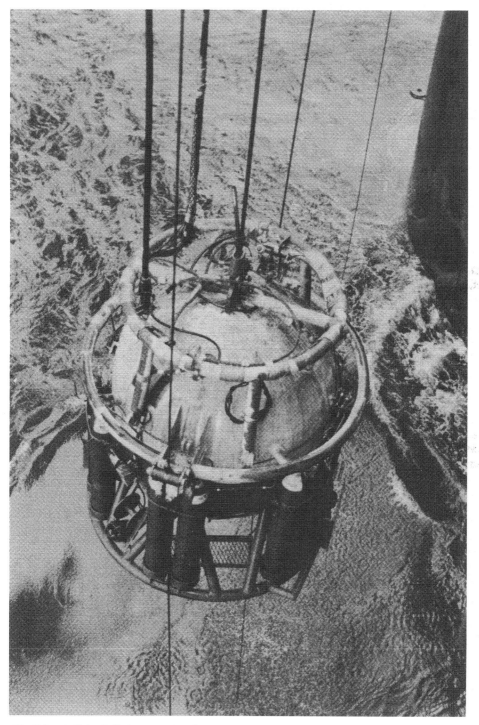

Fig. 7.3. A diving bell about to enter the water.

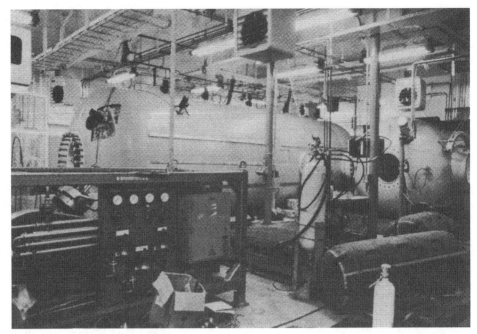

Fig. 7.4. A saturation decompression complex on the semisubmersible S.S. Sedco-Phillips.

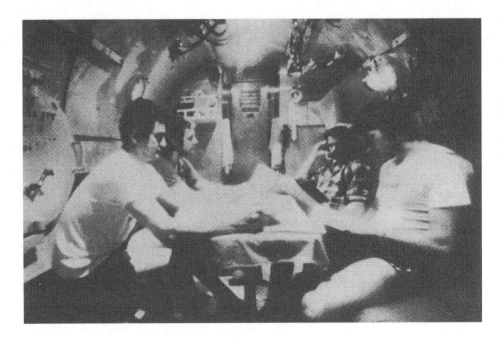

Fig. 7.5. Divers relaxing in the deck decompression chamber during a saturation dive.

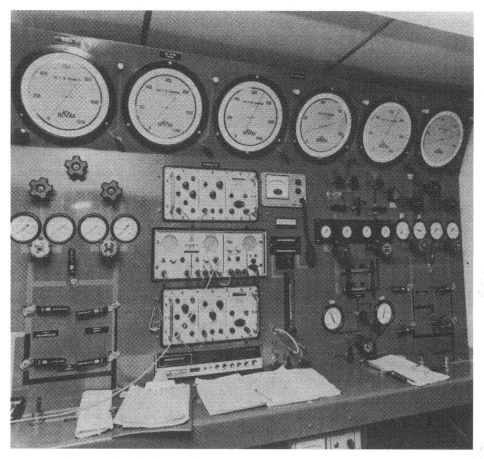

Fig. 7.6. The control panel of a saturation complex.

Gases Used in Diving

Air

Compressed air is still the most widely used breathing gas in commercial diving. In Britain it is only allowed for dives to a depth of 50 m, although in the United States the limit is 60 m. Beyond about 30 m, air is noticeably narcotic, and this is related to the amount of nitrogen which dissolves in the lipids of the nervous system. The symptoms closely resemble those seen in the induction of anaesthesia with nitrous oxide. Nitrogen is five times more soluble in fat than in water, and the gas content of the fatty areas of the brain and spinal cord predisposes them to decompression sickness. This risk increases with increasing depths and durations.

Mixed Helium and Oxygen (Heliox)

Helium is the ideal inert gas for diving, having almost the same solubility in water as in lipid. It also offers a low resistance to breathing and is not narcotic to depths in excess of 600 m, although at these extreme pressures it may be involved in the production of the tremor, microsleep and nausea known as the high-pressure nervous syndrome (HPNS). It has been shown to be helpful to include a small percentage of nitrogen in the mixture to reduce these symptoms, but this increases the subsequent risk of decompression sickness. Two other problems associated with the use of high-pressure heliox are voice distortion, which requires an unscrambler, and heat balance because of the combination of high thermal conductivity and capacity. Open sea diving trials have been undertaken to 500 m, but very few working dives have been made below 320 m.

The percentage of oxygen in air is, of course, fixed at 21%, giving, therefore, a fixed partial pressure of oxygen in compressed air at a given depth. Oxygen must be added to helium, and this allows the partial pressure to be varied. A minimum partial pressure of 0.18 bar is necessary to support an exercising diver, but it is usual for the level used to lie between 0.4 and 1.6 bar in saturation and bounce diving, respectively. Clearly, too low a partial pressure of oxygen causes unconsciousness to develop rapidly. In the case of pure helium it takes only a few breaths; the accidental inhalation of helium alone is so lethal it should not be stored or used at diving sites, for a 2% oxygen mixture can easily be substituted for dives to 200 m. For deeper dives a lower percentage is necessary. Although a partial pressure of oxygen above 3 bars may, over a period of time, cause the diver to convulse, providing the diver's breathing equipment is retained, and the diver does not drown, no harm will result. This is also a strong argument in favour of a helmet rather than a mask. In addition, over long periods oxygen has an irritant effect on the lungs, causing a progressive fall in vital capacity, an effect which is determined by a time-pressure relationship. A very small number of working dives have also been made to 190 m with a mixture of neon and oxygen and there has recently been a resurgence of interest in the use of hydrogen. Hydrogen has the advantage of being light, non-narcotic (though slightly euphoric) and cheap, but it has the great disadvantage of being explosive when mixed with oxygen which is likely to limit its commercial use.

Decompression Techniques

Decompression stoppages or 'stops' are needed to return the diver to atmospheric pressure if the 'no decompression' bottom times are exceeded. The 'no stop' bottom times are defined by the bounce dive curves for the particular gas breathed and are included in military manuals.

Decompression stops may be made either in the water or, if a bell is in use, in the bell or deck chamber. A technique called 'surface' decompression is also extensively used when the diver surfaces with or without stops and is recompressed in the deck chamber, breathing either air at 6.2 m or oxygen at 12 m (40 ft) before decompressing. Essentially, this technique involves an ascent with omitted decompression, with a recompression on the surface to treat any gas which has separated from solution. Hopefully this reduces the quantity of inert gas to levels which will not then give rise to symptoms.

A variety of techniques can be used to speed decompression in mixed gas bounce dives by changing the gases breathed during ascent. This is commonly done in deep short-duration dives where the decompression is long in relation to the working time on the bottom. Many different profiles are in use, some derived from military sources, while others, being proprietary information, are not available. The incidence of decompression sickness with these procedures is considerably higher than when saturation decompression procedures are used and includes serious cases, especially associated with a change from heliox to air.

Finally, saturation decompression times are very long, the most conservative being used by the US Navy, which uses an ascent rate of about 30 m per 24 h.

Medical Problems

Although the 'bends' or decompression sickness is the most widely known medical consequence of diving, many other problems occur more frequently on a commercial diving site. In fact, more accidents which involve loss of working time occur during work on deck than when divers are in the water. Accidents occurring to divers under pressure can be dealt with in a similar way to accidents to other personnel offshore, with two important exceptions. First, nitrous oxide must not be used to produce analgesia and second, the evacuation to shore must be as close to atmospheric pressure as possible. These factors are discussed in more detail later.

Work offshore is generally safer per unit cost than similar work onshore, even for surface workers. For example, fewer deaths and serious accidents occur in the construction of a major platform offshore than in a major civil engineering project onshore. This observation is especially true for divers, for they have a buoyant protective environment and a supply of carefully filtered breathing gas which eliminates the likelihood of occupational lung disease. Accidents in the water tend to be either relatively trivial, because the velocity of any moving object is reduced, or fatal because the diver is either asphyxiated or drowned.

Ear and Sinus Problems

It is a necessary prerequisite for commercial divers to be able to equalise middle ear pressure on descent; nevertheless, ear problems are still the largest single cause of morbidity in commercial diving. A *squeeze* occurs when, for example, the middle ear or a nasal sinus fails to equalise in pressure during compression because it is a rigid-walled cavity. The soft tissues are forced into the space, causing pain and often haemorrhage. In the case of the ear, the drum is forced into the middle ear and may rupture. If the ears clear unequally there may be stimulation of the semicircular canal otoliths which produces vertigo. Squeeze may also occur in relation to diving dress, for example in hard hat or helmet diving the diver may be forced into his helmet during descent by failing to equalise his suit pressure. Sometimes the pain of a limb-bend intensifies on recompression and it has been suggested that it is due to the tissues being squeezed into the gas cavity in the tissue. It is avoided or reduced by slowing the rate of recompression.

A reversed squeeze may occur on ascent if the gas contained in the middle ear cavity or sinuses cannot vent to ambient pressure. Both squeeze and reverse squeeze can occur when teeth contain gas cavities, usually associated with defective fillings.

Otitis externa occurs commonly when the meatus is constantly wet, which is another reason for the use of a helmet rather than a mask. Prophylactic drops are required in saturation diving because the high chamber humidity promotes the growth of gram-negative bacteria, especially *Pseudomonas aeruginosa*. A solution of aluminium acetate in 2% acetic acid is satisfactory when used twice a day. Should a florid infection occur, the treatment of choice is a mixture of polymyxin and gentamicin drops.

Middle ear infections are comparatively rare, but it is important to treat any perforation occurring on pressurisation vigorously with antibiotics and prohibit diving for at least 3 weeks.

Other Injuries in the Water or in Chambers

The hand is, of course, very vulnerable in any manual occupation and in diving a great deal of work is done by touch. Finger amputations are not uncommon, although they heal surprisingly well, but they and lacerations should be covered by antibiotics when available. Suturing under local anaesthesia presents no difficulty under pressure and crush injuries have been decompressed without any particular problem due to gas formation.

Near-Drowning

The inhalation of water may complicate any accident in the water and should not be forgotten in the management of diving accidents. It is dealt with in the section on drowning, together with hypothermia which may also complicate a diving accident (see pp. 98–106).

Pulmonary Barotrauma

Trauma to the lungs as a result of a rapid reduction of pressure is not uncommon in amateur diving, but is rare in commercial diving. This relates to the use of SCUBA and a mouth-piece in sport diving. In commercial diving the diver has a reserve supply in the event of the failure of the umbilical supply, and also has a residual volume of gas in the helmet or mask.

However, pulmonary barotrauma must always be considered when a diver makes an emergency ascent to surface for whatever reason. It is extremely rare in bell diving and chamber decompression because of the controlled rate of decompression. It is the rate of volume change close to the surface which is important. Death has followed the use of compressed air equipment in less than 2 m water. There are three complications possible, mediastinal 'surgical' emphysema, pneumothorax and arterial gas embolism. 'Surgical' emphysema alone does not require any treatment unless there is a respiratory obstruction or gas is trapped in the mediastinum when the diver is under pressure. The same is true for a pneumothorax, which is best resolved by the inhalation of oxygen at surface rather than the insertion of a chest tube. If a pneumothorax occurs in a diver under pressure, however, it is essential to insert a tube into the pleural cavity because of the expansion of the trapped gas causing a tension pneumothorax. A large-bore needle is all that is required to vent the excess gas during decompression, and there is usually little difficulty in deciding the correct side. It is very rare for mediastinal emphysema or pneumothorax to be complicated by the third complication of barotrauma, that is, gas embolism. Arterial gas embolism is thought to cause cardiac arrest by affecting the circulation through either the brain stem or the coronary arteries, but sudden death is fortunately very rare. More usually the diver loses consciousness or produces focal neurological signs within minutes of surfacing. The treatment is immediate recompression, and this will be dealt with in the section on treatment procedures.

Decompression Sickness

Although the importance of gas formation has frequently been questioned in the production of decompression sickness, there is no doubt that the separation of gas from solution is responsible for the initial symptoms. Bubbles only form when the gas is free in liquid. In tissues, the constraints of the various fascial planes determine the form and path taken by the gas. Gas phase forms because of significant reduction in the partial pressure of gas breathed relative to the gas in solution in the body. Normally this reduction is a result of a fall in the absolute pressure, that is decompression, but it can also result from a change in the inert gas concentration in the gas breathed, without a fall in the absolute pressure because of isobaric supersaturation.

The symptoms produced by the gas clearly relate to the site of formation. They have been classified by Haldane as types 1 and 2 and are referred to as 'simple' and 'serious'. It is important to recognise that there is *no progression implied* in this numbering. Deep air dives are much more likely in some schedules to produce serious rather than simple decompression sickness.

Type 1, or Simple Decompression Sickness

This is defined as a skin rash or pain in or around a joint. There is little debate about the mechanism of skin-bends, for bubbles have actually been observed in the lymphatics and blood vessels of the skin. The area shows a mottled appearance with areas of cyanosis and erythema. Normally itching is present.

Joint pain has been the subject of a great deal of academic discussion, but since it is not fatal, a certain amount of debate is inevitable. Nonetheless, it is highly significant that no pathology has ever been ascribed to the condition. After the demonstration by radiography of gas around the knee joint in aviators complaining of the 'bends', and the resolution of both the pain and gas on the radiographs during descent, there really are no grounds for believing it is anything other than a mechanical disruption of connective tissue by bubbles, a mechanism first suggested by Boycott, Damant and Haldane in 1908.

It is necessary to add a note of caution, however, about the description of this form of type 1 decompression sickness as being 'pain only', for neurological problems can produce pain. For example, spinal decompression sickness may present with atypical limb pains or girdle pain.

Type 2, or Serious Decompression Sickness

There are two categories of problem which have consequences involving the respiratory and nervous systems, respectively.

Respiratory decompression sickness may clearly relate to two factors: gas embolising the lung from the systemic venous return and gas actually forming in the tissues of the respiratory tract. These are likely to be inter-related and combine to give the dyspnoea and pain of the classic 'chokes'. The condition is usually associated with omitted decompression, but is seen occasionally following deep air dives. It may also be produced by a sudden change in the inert gas breathed during decompression.

Neurological decompression sickness may affect both the peripheral and central nervous systems. Parasthesiae are quite common during decompression from compressed air dives and may relate to either system. Evidence is rapidly accumulating that gas formation in the myelin, triggered by arterial microbubbles, is responsible for the disturbance of function. Because the blood flow to the white matter is so much larger in the brain than in the spinal cord, permanent lesions are much more common in the cord, particularly in the lower thoracic segments. But cerebellar and vestibular pathways have a relatively poor blood supply and are frequently involved, sometimes resulting in permanent damage. Visual disturbances are also fairly common, but it is extremely rare for any permanent loss of vision to result. The most common presentation is weakness in the legs and an inability to micturate. It would seem likely that gas formation may frequently occur in the myelin of the cord, but remains at sub-symptomatic levels. There is a considerable difference in the incidence of neurological decompression sickness between equivalent dives on air and heliox. It was first noticed in the US Navy, in 1938. When deep salvage was undertaken using heliox, no cases of unconsciousness or paralysis occurred, in marked contrast to the frequent problems associated with deep diving on compressed air. The reason for the difference relates to the fat solubility of the two gases. Nitrogen is about five times more soluble in fat than water and this relates to its ability to produce narcosis at high partial pressures, a condition identical to the induction of anaesthesia. A fundamental understanding of gas behaviour in the body is essential to a scientific approach to decompression and to the treatment of decompression sickness. The rate of gas movement is called the gas flux.

$$\text{Gas flux} = \text{Diffusion coefficient} \times \text{Solubility}$$

The diffusion coefficient and solubility must be defined for a given inert gas and for a given tissue. In fat, the flux of helium is only half that of nitrogen, whereas oxygen is twice as fast as nitrogen.

Treatment of Gas Embolism and Decompression Sickness

The objectives of treatment are the elimination of gas which has separated from solution and the relief of secondary effects like hypoxia, oedema and hypovolaemia. The basis of treatment is recompression, and generally the longer this is delayed the more difficult it becomes to achieve complete success.

In recent years there has been an increasing tendency to limit the depth used in treatment. This has derived from the difficulties encountered in using compressed air to resolve decompression sickness which has arisen from diving on the same gas. On recompression two effects occur:

1. A reduction in the volume of any gases present separated from solution
2. An increase in the partial pressure of the gases present in tissues and blood separated from solution

Both these effects are instantaneous, but the total resolution of the gas depends on its return into solution, which is dependent on effect 2, for the increased partial pressure of the gas present is entirely responsible for the elimination of the gaseous phase. The success of recompression can now be seen to lie in the under-saturation of the tissue and tissue fluid surrounding the separated gas on recompression. When the inert gas in the gas phase is nitrogen and the recompression is undertaken on air, it is clearly a race between the return of the gas into solution and the elevation of the inert gas content of the surrounding tissue from the perfusing blood, because of the raised partial pressure of nitrogen in the gas being breathed. This clearly introduces a quantitative aspect into what is usually regarded as a qualitative problem. In simple terms, if the number of gas molecules of nitrogen separated from solution is large and they cannot quickly be re-dissolved, then the gas phase is not likely to be easily eliminated when the recompression is undertaken breathing air, because of its nitrogen content.

This is one reason why the air recompression tables have not always been success-ful in the treatment of neurological decompression sickness, and have been super-seded by the 'shallow' oxygen tables. The recompression is limited to 18 m because of the danger of convulsions from oxygen toxicity. However, it is important to remember that any oxygen molecules remaining in gas phase after the metabolic demands of the tissue have been met will behave as an inert gas on decompression and may be responsible for mechanical effects. Circulating bubbles have been detected during the decompression phase of therapeutic tables. Oxygen has twice the flux of nitrogen in fat and twice the solubility.

Based on this data, the authors suggest the use of heliox for the treatment of embolism and type 2 decompression sickness in commercial diving. It is also indi-cated in some type 1 cases. Helium and oxygen are readily available, and helium has the lowest flux in body lipids and also the lowest resistance to breathing of the inert gases in commercial use. Unfortunately, opinion is currently moving in the opposite direction because of a misunderstanding of the phenomenon of gas counter-trans-port. Breathing air in a helium-and-oxygen environment is likely to lead to death. However, the opposite situation has not given rise to any difficulty, and has been used in commercial bell diving on a regular basis. There is good clinical evidence to support the use of helium-and-oxygen mixtures in treatment and the scientific data should eventually ensure its acceptance. For the moment it is necessary to review current practice and indicate the specific problem areas in therapy. An exhaustive description of the many problems which can arise is beyond the scope of this section, but the following comments may be useful.

Air Diving

Air Embolism

Standard Practice.   Immediate recompression to 50 m (165 ft) breathing air for at least 30 min (USN Table 6A), or 2 h (RN Table 54).

Problems.   The diver may have residual nitrogen present from the dive which caused the barotrauma, and this re-pressurisation on air may cause the emergence of serious decompression sickness on decompression. On the other hand, too rapid an ascent rate may cause the diver to embolise again and this will require further recompression. Gas embolism increases endothelial permeability and is used experi-mentally to disrupt blood–brain barrier function. It is important to utilise the vasoconstrictive action of elevated partial pressures of oxygen in the early hours of treatment. The utilisation of helium and oxygen mixtures allows the partial pressure of oxygen to be adjusted to about 2 atm to relieve hypoxia and control oedema and avoids the difficulties associated with nitrogen during decompression. Heliox also allows an indefinite stay at depth.

Decompression Sickness

Type 1

Standard Practice.   Oxygen at 18 m (60 ft) (USN Table 5, RN Table 61)

Problems.   Recurrences may occur after the shorter oxygen tables and divers may mis-diagnose spinal cord decompression sickness, presenting with pain as the initial symptom. Therefore at least use the longer oxygen tables (USN Table 6, RN Table 62)

Type 2

Standard Practice.   Oxygen at 18 m (60 ft) (USN Table 6, RN Table 62).

Problems.   Symptoms may not be relieved and indeed may worsen with oxygen. The USN and RN schedules only allow recompression to 50 m (165 ft) on air from this point. This is most unlikely to resolve the situation and heliox should be used with recompression to 50 m. The schedules of the US Navy allow the use of 80/20 heliox as a substitute for air in their treatment tables. However, a saturation mode can be adopted in most chambers by providing a carbon dioxide scrubber.
   This is possibly due to vasoconstriction, but oxygen counter-transport may also occur. The problems associated with oxygen in the treatment of decompression sickness are as follows:

Restriction of depth to 2.8 bar
Intermittent exposure to air
Limitation of duration of therapy
Vasoconstriction with reduced perfusion
Gas counter-transport?
Fire risk — BIBS required

Mixed Gas Diving

Decompression sickness occurring after a dive on mixed gases must only be treated using oxygen or a mixture of helium and oxygen. Air must *never* be used other than as a chamber pressurisation gas when oxygen is breathed.

Sub-Saturation or 'Bounce' Dives

Type 1.   If arising on the surface or shallower than 18 m on decompression, give oxygen at 18 m (60 ft) (USN Table 6, RN Table 62). For bends under pressure, resume original decompression after the 18 m (60 ft) section of the table. If arising deeper than 18 m (60 ft) during decompression, recompress to depth of relief on heliox (pO_2 1.5–2.0 bar) on BIBS; hold for 2 h then resume original decompression.

Type 2. Recompress to depth of relief breathing heliox only. If there is insufficient heliox available to pressurise the chamber then compressed air may be used and the heliox used via the BIBS. The exhaust of the BIBS should be into the chamber in order to create a Trimix atmosphere.

Problem. Bounce dive tables may involve several gas changes: detailed consideration is beyond the scope of this section. Specialist advice should be sought but the rule is always to use heliox in recompression.

Saturation Dives

Fortunately, serious decompression sickness is very rare in this form of diving, but may result from 'excursions' from storage pressures.

Type 1. If arising at surface or shallower than 18 m (60 ft) during decompression, use oxygen at 18 m (60 ft) (USN Table 6, RN Table 62). For the bends under pressure, resume original decompression after holding for 75 min at 60 ft.

Type 2. Recompression on heliox at depth of relief; hold for *at least* 24 h before resuming a saturation decompression. The rates which may be used are as follows, but careful note should be made of the condition of the patient and the ascent stopped and recompression undertaken if symptoms recur.

Deeper than 100 m	1.5 m/h
100–10 m	1 m/h
10 m to surface	0.5 m/h

The chamber atmosphere partial pressure of oxygen should be no greater than 0.6 bar and no less than 0.4 bar.

Omitted Decompression and Blowup on Mixed Gas Diving

Recompression must always be on heliox; *never* on air. When symptoms are present, recompression must be to a depth of relief or to the working depth of the chamber. This depth should be held for a minimum of 12 h and specialist advice sought.

Notes

1. In all cases of decompression sickness, but especially in serious cases, fluids should be used to ensure an adequate urine output. The ingestion or infusion of a fluid containing very little gas will result in a reduction of the size of circulating bubbles and the elimination of gas in urine. A chart of pulse rate and urine output should be kept.
2. Decompression must never be continued if the patient's condition worsens; depth is synonymous with safety in the treatment of decompression disorders and there is no benefit to be gained by hospitalisation.
3. A classic trap exists with unresolved symptoms at 50 m (165 ft) on air and after the maximum normal holding period of 2 h. Deeper compression is clearly needed, but current schedules only allow for decompression. Patients have been kept for up to 26 h at this depth before a saturation mode has been

arranged, but the recommended course is to establish a helium-and-oxygen atmosphere as soon as possible and recompress to the depth of relief or the maximum working depth of the chamber.

4. A trial of recompression is a valuable diagnostic tool which also has the merit of being therapeutic. If in doubt, recompress.

Immediate Treatment of Decompression Sickness when a Chamber is not on Site.

This situation rarely occurs in commercial diving, although delayed symptoms may sometimes occur when a diver has left the site of operations. It is more usual in amateur diving, particularly following repetitive dives. Unconsciousness in divers should be regarded as being due to air embolism until proven otherwise.

Air Embolism

This problem is a more frequent cause of morbidity and mortality in amateur diving than decompression sickness. Initial resuscitation may include artificial respiration, 100% oxygen and intravenous fluids. It is essential to transport the patient to a recompression chamber with the minimum delay. Patients have occasionally made a spectacular recovery from a moribund state with delays of up to 26 h. When helicopters and non-pressurised aircraft are used, they should fly at the minimum altitude consistent with safety.

Type 1
Skin rashes are likely to clear spontaneously over a period, but care should be taken to ensure that no neurological abnormality is present; 100% oxygen breathing and oral fluids should be used when available. Joint pain can be treated by analgesics together with oxygen and oral fluids. Normally pain will resolve in 24 h.

Type 2
Respiratory distress should be treated with 100% oxygen and again fluids should be used, but ideally should be given intravenously. Transport should be arranged to the nearest recompression facility by the fastest means possible. Where aircraft are used, the cabin pressure should be as close to 1 bar as possible. If a portable recompression chamber is available, then the patient may be transported under pressure to a definitive care facility.

Professional Bodies Associated with Diving

There are a number of professional bodies, societies and committees which are concerned with the medical aspects of diving. Some of these are open for membership by any doctor who is interested in diving medicine, but most are professional committees which are prepared to advise on particular topics. A list of these organisations and the addresses at which they can be contacted appears in Appendix 5.

Medical Examination of Divers

Most diving companies, regardless of the statutory arrangements in force in the countries in which they are operating, require a diver to possess a medical certificate of fitness to dive, for insurance purposes. Some countries, for example Britain and Norway, require a statutory examination of fitness. Very often this statutory examination serves also to satisfy the diving company, but this can lead to a degree of conflict, for example in some cases of bone necrosis, where the doctor may feel that a diver may continue, but his employer may not accept any diver with a lesion.

It is not necessary for an examining doctor to be a diving medical specialist in order for him to determine whether or not a person is fit to dive, but he should have a good knowledge and understanding of diving, diving techniques and the physiological demands made upon the diver in the course of his work. The doctor should have attended one of the recognised basic courses in hyperbaric medicine. Conversely, a doctor who may be totally competent to examine divers is not necessarily competent to undertake the care of a diver in a hyperbaric emergency situation. In the United Kingdom and Norway, medical practitioners have to be approved by the Health and Safety Executive (Petroleum Directorate, Norway) before they can issue medical certificates of fitness to dive under the Diving Operations at Work Regulations (1981).

One popular misconception is that saturation diving on mixed gas is more dangerous. This is quite untrue. In relation to the number of hours spent in the water offshore, surface-orientated air diving is very much more dangerous and demands greater physical fitness.

The detail required in the statutory examinations varies from country to country, but it is essentially the same as any other thorough examination. The form of the examination, in the United Kingdom, is currently being reviewed by a working party of the Health and Safety Executive.

The current forms (MS74) to be used for the recording of clinical data are, in the opinion of the authors, totally inadequate. However, it is expected that better, more comprehensive data sheets will be issued with the new HSE MAI booklet *The Medical Examination of Divers*. It is hoped that examining doctors will retain the clinical data safely and indefinitely. With the closure of the Medical Research Council Decompression Sickness Registry, there is no longer any central depository for the collection of these data, a source of much regret to the industry. In future any comparison of clinical data, either for purposes of assessment or epidemiological review will be dependent upon examining doctors retaining and making available their clinical records.

The medical examination of divers must be comprehensive, detailed, and so conducted that a diver returning from his annual examination can be fully confident of his own physical capability to do his job. The purpose of the examination is to determine whether the person is physically and psychologically fit and also to establish the current medical status of the diver to produce a baseline against which any future medical changes can be compared.

In addition to the normal medical instruments required to perform a physical examination, the following apparatus is needed by a physician who intends to perform regular medical examinations on divers:

1. Electrocardiograph
2. Harpenden skinfold callipers
3. Audiometer

4. A wedge bellows spirometer (e.g. Vitalograph)
5. Access to radiological and pathology facilities for the performance of long bone and chest X-rays and blood tests

Some numerically quantifiable test for the measurement of physical fitness is helpful. There are various exercise tolerance tests, but a candidate must not fail to pass the following simple test — after stepping up on a chair five times in 5 s, the pulse should return to the pre-exercise rate in 45 s. A test which gives a numerical result expressed as a percentage has been used regularly by the authors and is as follows.

The patient is asked to step up and down onto a 50 cm chair at the rate of 30 times per minute for a total of 5 min or until exhausted, whichever is sooner. The man lies down immediately and his pulse rate is recorded over three separate periods of 30 s: after 30 s rest, after 2 min rest and after 4 min rest. The rating of physical fitness is then calculated as follows:

$$\frac{t \times 100}{p \times 2}$$

where t is the time taken to complete the exercise in seconds and p is the sum of the three post-exercise pulse counts.

The result can be assessed as follows:

Below 41, unfit
41–74, average
75–90, good
Over 90, excellent

As with any other test of physical fitness this provides only a very rough and ready guide, but when it is repeated annually it does allow comparisons to be made. The test also stimulates a valuable competitive spirit among divers who therefore strive to achieve the maximum standard of physical fitness.

Physical Standards

Age

There is no upper age limit for divers as long as all the medical standards are met though, in practice, few divers continue in their professional careers over the age of 40.

Stature

The diver must be physically robust and not carrying excessive fat. Skinfold measurements will distinguish the fat person from the muscular one.

Skin

The constant wetness experienced by divers and the high humidity of saturation chambers are particularly threatening to skin compromised by trauma or disease. Almost any active skin disease is a contraindication to diving.

Ears

There should be no history of ear disease and the diver must be able to clear his ears. Disease of the middle ear such as chronic infection, 'glue ear' or a perforated tympanic membrane are causes for rejection. Chronic or acute otitis externa is also a contraindication. Otitis externa can become florid and totally disabling in a compression chamber. Hearing should be assessed audiometrically, but the diver must be able to hear and understand normal conversation unaided.

Respiratory System

A chest X-ray is certainly required at the initial examination. Thereafter the decision is left to the discretion of the examining doctor but most diving physicians would perform an annual chest X-ray. Some respiratory conditions will preclude diving. These include any respiratory infection, sarcoid, pneumonitis, lung cysts, emphysematous blebs and bullae, pneumothorax, pleural effusion, lung fistula, bronchiectasis, fibrosis or malignancy. Chronic bronchitis, emphysema or asthma will also disqualify as will a history of spontaneous pneumothorax. A history of childhood asthma is not necessarily a contraindication as long as there is now normal lung function and no evidence, on formal testing, of bronchoconstriction brought on by exertion, lung irritants or cold inhalation. A history of pneumothorax provoked by unusual respiratory stress or following surgery may be compatible with diving as long as 3 months have elapsed to allow healing and if full functional investigation shows no evidence of local or generalised airflow obstruction. The same considerations apply following thoracic trauma. Respiratory function must be assessed using a wedge bellows spirometer and the values for forced vital capacity and forced expired volume in one second recorded. The predicted values for these parameters can be obtained from the following formulae:

FVC	Male	$5.2 \times H - 0.022 \times A - 3.60$ (SD 0.58)
	Female	$5.2 \times H - 0.018 \times A - 4.36$ (SD 0.44)
FEV_1	Male	$3.7 \times H - 0.028 \times A - 1.59$ (SD 0.52)
	Female	$3.29 \times H - 0.029 \times A - 1.42$ (SD 0.36)

Where A is the age in years and H is the height in metres. A value more than one standard deviation below the mean should be fully investigated at a respiratory laboratory.

Cardiovascular System

The cardiovascular system must be normal to palpation and auscultation and the resting blood pressure should not exceed 140/90, taking the fifth phase as the indicator. An ECG before and after symptom-limited exercise should always be performed at the initial examination and, thereafter, at the discretion of the examining doctor.

Any organic heart disease will be a cause for rejection as will coarctation of the aorta and any evidence of coronary insufficiency or myocardial ischaemia. Coronary artery bypass surgery will not render a person fit for diving. Disorders of rhythm or ECG abnormalities should be referred for cardiological assessment and will usually be a cause for rejection unless demonstrably benign. Hypertension requiring therapy is a cause for rejection and also cardiomegaly, except for those divers with athletic hearts confirmed by a cardiologist.

Alimentary System

Chronic inflammatory bowel disease, malabsorptive conditions, hernias, acute or chronic hepatic dysfunction, gallstones, a history of pancreatitis, symptomatic hiatus hernia, active peptic ulceration and the presence of a stoma are all a bar to diving. Relative contraindications, each of which must be considered on its merits are, distal colitis or proctitis, recurrent abdominal pain, reflux oesophagitis and haemorrhoids.

Genitourinary System

The presence of kidney stones is a cause for rejection as well as active venereal disease or blood or protein in the urine, unless orthostatic.

Endocrine System

Diabetes is a cause for rejection, while glycosuria will need full investigation. A proven or suspected endocrine abnormality will require specialised assessment.

Musculoskeletal System

Any diver must have unimpeded mobility. Recurrent episodes of incapacitating back pain will be a cause for rejection; in assessing divers with back problems it should be remembered that a diver may have to perform a lot of heavy lifting when he is out of the water. A diver may be declared fit after spinal surgery if the neurological examination is normal and full mobility regained. Routine long bone X-rays are no longer required, but X-rays of specific joints, usually shoulders, may be clinically indicated for a variety of reasons.

Central Nervous System

A detailed examination of all modalities of the nervous system is very important and must be fully recorded for comparison with any subsequent changes. A history of severe motion sickness or claustrophobia is an obvious reason for disqualification at the initial examination. Other historical reasons for barring a diver are unprovoked loss of consciousness, recurring fainting episodes or epilepsy after the age of 5, or severe migraine accompanied by sensory or motor disturbances. A history of any other neurological disorder will be an indication for further investigation, and particular attention should be paid to a history of recent head injury with the possibility of post-traumatic epilepsy.

Psychiatric Illness

Any evidence of past or present psychiatric disorder, including alcohol or drug abuse, should be a cause for rejection unless it was only of a very minor nature. A psychological assessment is particularly important at the initial examination.

Vision

Corrected vision should be at least 6/9 and N5 for near vision. Colour vision should be tested at the initial examination and the result entered in the diver's logbook.

Blood

A full blood count and test for sickle cell trait should be performed at the initial examination. Presence of sickle cell trait is a cause for rejection. The haemoglobin should be not less that 12 g and any disorder of bone marrow function likely to cause anaemia, haemolysis or a tendency to bleeding or clotting is a cause for rejection.

Female Divers

The same general standards apply to both male and female divers, but any female who considers that she may be pregnant should not dive.

Results of Examination

At the conclusion of the examination the results should be entered on the HSE medical record which should be completed in conjunction with the MAI document *The Medical Examination of Divers*. The result of the examination must also be entered in the diver's logbook, as prescribed by the Regulations. If an examining doctor finds a diver to be unfit or restricted in some way (e.g. to depth, time or a particular type of diving), the logbook must be appropriately endorsed. In these circumstances the diver should also be reminded that he may appeal for a review of his case to the Director of Medical Services of the Health and Safety Executive within 28 days.

Return to Diving Following Decompression Sickness and Other Illnesses

There has been considerable debate on this topic in recent years, with grossly conflicting views expressed. In commercial diving, companies generally have a written policy for insurance purposes, usually based on naval practices. However, it has become increasingly obvious that military practice is unduly conservative and not realistic in commercial diving, where action taken would be likely to terminate the employment of a diver on an offshore contract and thus lead to concealment of symptoms. This obviously will not serve the best interests of either the diver or his company. On the other hand, it is fair to point out that the risks that may be involved in diving, particularly deep air diving, are several orders of magnitude greater than those in most other occupations.

After Type 1 Decompression Sickness

A logical approach to simple decompression sickness must take into account the confirmation by ultrasound of Haldane's original observation that gas must form during most decompressions. The difference therefore between a diver who has decompression sickness and one who has not, after the same dive, is not likely to relate to a large difference in the amount of gas present. It is likely to be due to the retention of a small amount of gas at a particular site which forms a critical volume and gives rise to symptoms. Following the resolution of the symptoms by the use of oxygen after a therapeutic compression, the diver will surface after a trial by decompression with very much less inert gas in his body than his colleague who has not developed the symptoms. The normal minimum period between dives allowed by the navies, to avoid the constraints of a repetitive dive, is 12 h. It is therefore reasonable to double this minimum period before the next dive following simple decompression sickness. However, an air diver could immediately enter a saturation dive which would be excellent treatment, but the converse, that is, a mixed gas diver undertaking an air dive, must *not* be permitted under the 12 h.

After Type 2 Decompression Sickness

Respiratory decompression sickness, or the 'chokes', is now almost unknown in mixed gas bounce diving and there is no case in the literature where it has followed a mixed gas saturation dive. However, it still occurs in air diving, although it responds very rapidly to recompression on oxygen. Because of the possibility of temporary impairment of the lung's ability to filter bubbles, it would seem reasonable for the minimum period on the surface to be 48 h.

Neurological decompression sickness can be divided into two categories, first, where there is no obvious disability, and second, where objective evidence is present. It is clearly desirable for divers to report symptoms early, particularly where the nervous system is involved, but there is a natural reluctance to do so and this is greatly increased if the penalty in terms of loss of employment is considerable. On this basis it would seem reasonable to divide the presentation of decompression sickness into three categories:

1. The diver reports symptoms, but there is little associated disability and the problem is rapidly resolved on recompression. It is recommended that the surface interval after treatment should be about 48 h for further air or mixed gas bounce dives, although it may be omitted entirely for a heliox saturation pressurisation.

2. Symptoms which are accompanied by obvious disability resolved by treatment and where the diver is fit on surfacing. The interval on the surface should be at least 5 days, and specialist advice should be obtained before any attempt is made to transfer the diver to shore.

3. Cases where there is evidence or doubt that the condition has been resolved offshore. The diver should be recompressed and specialist advice sought immediately.

Flying After Diving

As a general rule flying should be avoided for 24 h after any diving and 48 h after diving below 50 m or saturation diving. If flying is essential, the flight should be delayed for as long as possible after the dive and the aircraft should fly as low as is compatible with safety. In a pressurised aircraft the cabin pressure should be kept as near to atmospheric as possible. Following treatment for decompression sickness a period of *at least* 48 h should be allowed to elapse before flying in any type of aircraft.

Transport of a Patient with Decompression Sickness

All cases of decompression sickness or air embolism should be transferred to the nearest recompression facility as soon as possible. Even after a considerable delay in treatment, hyperbaric therapy, particularly with oxygen, can produce dramatic improvement. Every diving supervisor must know the location of the nearest recompression chamber and the quickest means of reaching it, along with the telephone numbers of diving medical specialists that he can contact. When an ambulance is used to transport a person with decompression sickness it should, if possible, allow him to stand up. If he is conscious, the patient should be transported in the supine position, and in a three-quarter prone position if he is unconscious. In either case, the head should be kept slightly lower than the rest of the body. Oxygen should be continuously administered, but nitrous oxide analgesia is definitely contraindicated and should never be used on a patient with suspected decompression sickness.

Transport by air is ideally accomplished in a helicopter which can fly at an altitude not exceeding 300 m and if possible, should endeavour to keep below 150 m. Where transport of the patient has to be by sea, then the fastest available craft should be used. Time may be saved by arranging a rendezvous with another faster boat such as a lifeboat in the United Kingdom, or a coastguard cutter in the United States, and transferring the casualty to speed the journey, or it may be possible to rendezvous with a vessel carrying a compression chamber.

In all cases, a medical attendant should accompany the patient and it is a wise precaution to set up an intravenous infusion before commencing the journey. This will maintain the patient's fluid balance, enable plasma expanders to be given if necessary and also facilitate the intravenous administration of drugs. Dehydration and haemoconcentration are problems in all cases of decompression sickness, and the conscious patient should be encouraged to drink an adequate amount of fluid.

Transfer Under Pressure and Hyperbaric Rescue

Over the past few years, many hours have been spent discussing the requirement for the rescue of divers from the hyperbaric environment. The issue has been somewhat confused by trying to consider both the main indications for hyperbaric rescue in the same context. Divers may need to be rescued when they are in a saturation complex on a rig which has to be evacuated for one reason or another, and it may also be necessary to remove a sick or injured diver from a saturation unit. Most hyperbaric rescue systems are based upon a portable 'flyaway' chamber which can be locked onto the chamber offshore, transported by helicopter and mated with a special 'medical' compression chamber onshore. There are certain inherent problems in this type of system. First, there is no universal mating flange, so some form of adaptor is also required for all chambers which are not compatible. Second, the portable chamber is rarely large enough to hold more than two people and it may not be possible to gain access to them during transport. Third, there are technical problems and some dangers in handling a compression chamber with two people inside. Fourth, there are problems of maintaining life support during transit.

In view of these difficulties and dangers one may ask what advantages are to be gained. In the case of the sick diver the most important is that he can be moved to a place where there is more expert assistance and better medical facilities. Also, the actual diving operation can continue without interruption, which may be a very substantial consideration in terms of cost. On the other hand, the very high cost of providing an emergency hyperbaric rescue system for the very few occasions when it may be needed cannot be justified on economic grounds alone.

If the transfer under pressure system is also used for training and research, to defray some of the cost, it cannot and should not be required to be immediately available when it is required in an emergency, because the patient offshore must be fully stabilised before a transfer is attempted and this will take some time.

During the history of the exploration and development of the North Sea, there have been only two incidents in which the transfer under pressure system may have been useful if it had been available. (Since this was written the system has been used effectively and successfully on at least one occasion.) On all other occasions when a diver has required medical assistance under pressure, it has been provided by taking to the site a doctor or doctors who have attended the patient in the chamber on the rig or barge.

It seems to us that the provision of a trained, skilled mobile medical team, as described elsewhere in this book, who can render first aid and maintain the condition of the patient until he can be removed from the chamber and transported to hospital, is the best insurance in this sort of situation, and much preferable to transferring the patient ashore under pressure.

Furthermore, a transfer under pressure system is very unlikely to be of any use in the evacuation of a saturation system in the event of a rig or barge catching fire or breaking up in bad weather. In these circumstances, some form of hyperbaric lifeboat, with all the dangers which are associated with it, is the only hope of survival which the trapped divers may have.

Sources of Assistance in a Diving Emergency

Any doctor may occasionally find himself confronted by a hyperbaric problem, perhaps in a diver with decompression sickness in a chamber, or a patient with symptoms which he believes could be due to decompression sickness. In either case, the average doctor with no experience in this field would welcome the opportunity to obtain expert help.

The Royal Navy have traditionally provided this sort of expertise, but they have not enough manpower to meet the demands which would be made upon them if they alone had to take care of the medical problems of modern commercial diving in the United Kingdom and elsewhere. Even so, the Royal Navy never fail to provide help whenever they are requested.

Many diving companies have their own medical officers who are skilled and experienced in hyperbaric medicine and indeed, in some cases, have been instrumental in formulating the medical standards and techniques by which modern diving is conducted. They have made an immense contribution, but, from a practical point of view, they may not always be available when required in an emergency or, because of distance or language, communications may be very difficult. Several academic institutions, especially in the United States, have hyperbaric facilities and experienced staff who are happy to proffer advice.

Two organisations at the main centres of offshore exploration in the United Kingdom, Great Yarmouth and Aberdeen, have experts in underwater medicine and operate on a 24 h basis. In addition there are several physicians in private practice who have acquired an expertise in diving medicine.

Many of the oil companies have physicians within their medical departments who are experts in diving medicine. A full list of these possible sources of assistance in an emergency appears in Appendix 13.

Long-term Effects of Diving

Shallow-water diving has been practised since Alexander descended in a diving bell, the Kolympha, in about 330 B.C. A Frenchman by the name of Freminet was the first to use compressed air to supply the diver in the water, but Augustus Siebe was the first person to develop a diving dress using compressed air and an exhaust valve. However until the 1960s, diving for practical purposes was limited to about 50 m. Even then, no experimental or epidemiological work was done to ascertain any possible long-term effects of repeated exposure to a hyperbaric environment. Aseptic necrosis of bone in tunnel workers was first described by Bassoe (1911) in the United States and Bornstein and Plate in Germany (1911–1912). There is little doubt now that the development of this condition is related to hyperbaric exposure, but the mechanism by which it occurs is still not clear. The incidence appears, however, to be related more to the number of decompressions than to the total time of exposure to pressure. The first case of aseptic bone necrosis in a diver was described in 1941. Since then the decompression sickness panel of the Medical Research Council have recorded 65 juxta-articular lesions from 5110 men in their registry at Newcastle-upon-Tyne. But up to now this is the only proven adverse health effect of diving.

It should not be assumed that, because this is so, no others can be expected. Deep diving has not yet been practised long enough, nor have the numbers involved been great enough for epidemiological studies to have much meaning, though some centres have now accumulated sufficient data to enable some preliminary surveys to be undertaken.

On theoretical grounds one might seek long-term changes in lungs, heart or metabolism. Crosbie et al. (1977) looked at the lungs of 404 North Sea divers and found no significant abnormalities. Divers who commence their diving careers before the age of 20 appear to develop large lungs, but there is no real evidence that they develop emphysema as was at one time suggested. Following incidental findings of some moderate right ventricular hypertrophy in a small series of autopsies, Calder suggested that right ventricular strain may be a sequel of long hyperbaric exposure, but examination of a series of ECGs did not confirm any such effect, and he has not confirmed his original findings in a much larger and subsequent series of autopsies.

The same investigator has, however, shown that there may be extensive areas of damage to the spinal cord in some divers who, apparently, have no history of type 2 decompression sickness. This raises the question of 'silent' damage, such as infarction, occurring without clinical symptoms. This work and some anecdotal experiences related by the wives of divers to psychological investigators, along with a more general concern by the Norwegian authorities led to a symposium being held in Stavanger, Norway in November 1983 on the subject of *The Long-Term Neurological Consequences of Deep Diving*. This meeting was organised by the European Underwater Biomedical Society and the Norwegian Petroleum Directorate and its proceedings were published (EUBS-NPD 1983). As one would expect, no firm conclusions were reached at the meeting, but sufficient evidence was produced and some anxiety engendered among the participants, regarding the long-term effects, that 'there should be increased monitoring of divers to provide information which can be used as the base for future discussion'.

Various metabolic changes have been reported in association with saturation diving, including increased diuresis, retention of sodium, calcium and chloride, and an increased diuresis of potassium and phosphorus. Corticosteroid excretion has also been noticed to rise. These however appear to correct spontaneously on return to atmospheric pressure. Doran et al. (1985) have demonstrated disturbances in the level of glycoproteins which, they postulate, may be due to liver dysfunction. They further suggest that there may be a relationship between the liver dysfunction and the high-pressure nervous syndrome.

Since it has taken the human organism several million years to adapt to survival at an atmospheric pressure of 1 bar it would seem to be unlikely, on purely biological grounds, that it can be subjected to a profound change of pressure for long periods without producing some unfavourable changes. On these grounds alone, therefore, a close watch should be kept for early changes on those divers who are regularly working in saturation.

Drugs Under Pressure

This subject may be considered under three headings:

1. The use or misuse of addictive drugs
2. The incidental use of drugs in diving
3. The use of drugs in decompression sickness and other dysbaric disorders

The Use or Misuse of Addictive Drugs

The hallucinogens drastically affect mood and cause perceptual disorders. Some, such as LSD may cause 'panic reactions' and 'flashbacks'. Marijuana is also hallucinogenic and chronic use may lead to ocular damage and permanent functional changes in the brain. There is also anecdotal evidence that nitrogen narcosis potentiates the effect of cannabis dangerously, which is thought to have been a factor in several sport SCUBA diving accidents.

Nitrogen will also potentiate the analgesic effects of the opiates. The amphetamines, apart from being stimulants, also cause anxiety, psychoses and hallucinations. At times they can produce violent behaviour and methylamphetamine is known to cause cardiac dysrhythmias, an effect which may be potentiated by high levels of catecholamines which are released under stress or a raised partial pressure of carbon dioxide.

Cocaine causes CNS stimulation and an increased perceptual awareness, especially of an increased capacity for muscular work. Nitrogen narcosis will potentiate CNS depression which follows the stimulation by cocaine. Nitrogen will also potentiate the effects of any CNS depressants, including alcohol, barbiturates, benzodiazepines and methaqualone.

The use of any of this group of drugs is, therefore, incompatible with hyperbaric exposure. There is no situation, under pressure, either in the water or out of it, where any such drugs could be taken without compromising safety. Owing to their potential for causing flashbacks, there is a strong argument for permanently prohibiting diving to anyone who has ever taken one of the hallucinogens, such as LSD or mescaline.

The Incidental Use of Drugs in Diving

In this category we include all those drugs which may be needed to treat incidental illnesses unassociated with the hyperbaric exposure. The action of a drug may be affected by: (a) the inert gas; (b) the raised partial pressure of oxygen; (c) the pressure per se.

Pressure alone may affect the fluidity and order of lipoprotein biological membranes. It may also induce configurational change in proteins, so affecting their functions, and pressure acts at multiple sites in the CNS. Anaesthetics also appear to act at multiple sites and some of the sites of action of pressure may coincide complementarily or antagonistically with the sites of action of anaesthetics.

Pressure also exerts pharmacological effects outside the CNS such as the bradycardia induced in the heart. Practolol and atropine appear to prevent this effect. It would seem to be wise to exercise caution in using drugs which affect the autonomic innervation of the heart, under pressure. Many of the effects have only been demonstrated at very high pressures, but the effects are unlikely to have an absolute threshold. Some changes probably take place at the lower pressures encountered in commercial diving.

All inert gases have anaesthetic potency, with the exception of helium and hydrogen. Some anaesthetic agents bind to specific sites in myoglobin and haemoglobin. It is known that these proteins are also affected by inert gases and so the drug effects will be modified by inert gases at raised partial pressure, even at low dosages. Many other drugs, apart from those commonly used as anaesthetics, have anaesthetic properties and should, therefore, be used with extra care in the hyperbaric environment. These would include barbiturates, hypnotics, minor and major tranquillisers, antihistamines, motion sickness remedies, anti-nausea drugs and antidepressants.

Most drugs seem to react with hyperbaric oxygen, some exacerbating oxygen and some ameliorating it. Those which exacerbate it include dexamphetamine, epinephrine, norepinephrine, ephedrine, morphine and fentanyl. Those which ameliorate it include propanolol, anaesthetics, chlorpromazine, disulfiram, GABA, ganglion blockers, glutathione, reserpine, vitamin E, lithium, Hydergine, papaverine, serotonin, phenytoin, phenobarbitone, diazepam, aspirin and indomethacin. Perhaps the widespread interactions are not surprising since it is known that oxygen is capable of both enzyme inhibition and induction.

The effect of oxygen on the blood–brain barrier is conflicting and may vary from one substance to another. This is of marked importance in the hyperbaric environment; when the blood–brain permeability is increased, drugs which do not normally reach the brain may do so in varying amounts. The effects may be beneficial or harmful, depending upon the drug.

It is clearly impossible to evaluate the behaviour of every potential drug that we may wish to use under pressure, but some work has been done. For example, at 180 m (600 ft), the anti-inflammatory properties of cortisone were identical to what they were at sea level, as judged by histological changes and serum haptoglobin levels. Pain thresholds were modified by morphine analgesia at 19 atm in exactly the same way as at the surface. The LD_{50} for phenobarbitone, lignocaine, ethanol and histamine in hyperbaric heliox at 19 atm were the same as at sea level. The narcotic effects of nitrogen appear to be exacerbated by alcohol and ameliorated by amphetamine. The distribution of radioactively labelled penicillin in rats was similar at atmospheric pressure and at 21 atm, though there was a 20% increase in the mean brain concentration. Hyperbaric exposure to 12 atm heliox attenuated the development of ethanol tolerance in mice and the effects of ethanol, octanol and atropine in modifying neuromuscular transmission of frog end-plates are affected differently by pressure.

At a more practical level, a large number of diving physicians have pooled their experiences in the use of common drugs under pressure. Dexamethasone and aspirin have been used extensively and effectively under pressure. Pentazocine has been used to 50 m (170 ft) in heliox with fewer side effects than are often encountered at atmospheric pressure.

Considerable experience in the use of antibiotics has now been accumulated and no problems have been encountered with any of them. They seem to be equally effective at pressure as on the surface.

Experience with antihistamines confirms their complementary narcotic effect with nitrogen under pressure and they should be administered with special caution. Many readily obtainable, proprietary cough and cold remedies contain antihistamines.

Anti-inflammatory drugs such as ibuprofen and fenbufen seem to be safe and effective at normal dosage.

In conclusion, therefore, drugs in the hyperbaric environment should be administered with great caution and, if a diver is already taking a drug, he should not be allowed under pressure except in very special circumstances. However, in spite of the considerable caution which is necessary, no medication should be withheld in a serious or life-threatening situation because its effect under pressure may be undetermined. If the diver's condition demands a particular drug to save his life it should be given in the same dosage and the same manner as if he were on the surface. In our present state of knowledge it is not justified to withhold treatment.

The Use of Drugs as Adjuvant Therapy in Decompression Sickness

The following drugs may, from time to time, be used in the management of decompression sickness:

Normal saline
Dextran
Steroids
Heparin
Aspirin
Diazepam
Bronchodilators
Vasodilators
Anti-inflammatory drugs

Normal Saline

In moderate and severe cases of decompression sickness, loss of circulating blood volume is a significant factor and may lead to hypovolaemic shock. While colloid solutions have always been the traditional treatment, these are not without danger and it would therefore seem sensible to commence fluid replacement therapy with normal saline. One may administer 7 l saline over a period of 2–3 h without fear of complications and without prejudice to the subsequent administration of a colloid solution.

Dextran

Low molecular weight dextran will increase circulating blood volume, decrease 'sludging' and reduce platelet adhesiveness. Dextran 70 is probably preferable to dextran 40 because it remains longer in the circulation, it is excreted more slowly and it is less likely to traverse damaged capillaries.

However, dextran can cause sensitivity and anaphylactic reactions as well as kidney damage. Although it may have a valuable role in many difficult type 2 cases of decompression sickness it is advisable to exercise caution in its use and employ simpler solutions such as saline or Ringer's solution first.

Steroids

While there is still some controversy over the use of steroids in type 2 decompression sickness and gas embolism, they are regularly used with benefit in other conditions associated with cerebral oedema such as brain tumours and closed head injuries. Their regular use in cerebral decompression sickness and gas embolism is, therefore, based on well-established practice and most diving physicians would use them in these serious cases. When they are used, they should be administered intravenously and in large doses, e.g. methylprednisolone 2 g over 10 min or dexamethasone 4 mg every 6 h. They should be rapidly tailed off after 48–72 h.

Heparin

In high doses heparin prevents coagulation and, in lower doses, venous thrombosis. But the control of dosage is critical and not easy to achieve, even in hospital. It is extremely difficult in the circumstances in which decompression sickness is usually being treated and, in spinal cord decompression sickness, it may precipitate haemorrhage from an end-artery in an already compromised vascular situation. There is little evidence to support the use of heparin except, perhaps, in generalised intravascular coagulation.

Aspirin

Some physicians have used aspirin in the treatment of decompression sickness for many years because of its effect in preventing platelet aggregation. Aspirin is currently enjoying some popularity as a prophylactic agent in the prevention of coronary thrombosis, but the dosage for its use in this role is critical.

Aspirin acetylates and thereby inactivates the enzyme cyclo-oxygenase, which is responsible for the synthesis of thromboxane A2 which induces platelet aggregation and vasoconstriction in platelets. However, the same substance in vascular endothelium is responsible for the synthesis of prostacyclin which inhibits platelet aggregation and prompts vasodilatation. The antithrombotic effect of aspirin is thought to be due to its effect on platelet thromboxane A2 and it would appear that vascular endothelial prostacyclin synthesis is less susceptible to aspirin inhibition than the synthesis of platelet thromboxane A2. In theory, therefore, the optimal dose of aspirin is that which will inhibit thromboxane A2 synthesis, but does not affect prostacyclin synthesis. A single dose of 325 mg aspirin seems to affect both processes, but a dose of 100 mg or less only inhibits thromboxane A2 synthesis. If aspirin is used in decompression sickness, therefore, it would appear to be necessary to use much lower dosages, e.g. a single daily dose of 100 mg.

Diazepam

Some physicians have used diazepam routinely for the treatment of decompression sickness. Its benefits are probably indirect in relieving the anxiety which always accompanies decompression sickness. At least it is safe to use under pressure and may be helpful.

Bronchodilators

These drugs should only be used when there is severe wheezing and impaired gas exchange. Their administration may, however, facilitate the transpulmonic passage of gas bubbles from the venous to the arterial side of the circulation and these drugs should only be considered if there is severe bronchospasm, in which case aminophylline would appear to be safe to use under pressure.

Vasodilators

Though these drugs have been used frequently by some physicians, there is no evidence that they have any benefit in decompression sickness.

Anti-inflammatory Drugs

This group of drugs, like aspirin, also inactivate the enzyme cyclo-oxygenase which may be the explanation for the benefit observed from their administration in decompression sickness. Ibuprofen and dicloferal have both been used effectively.

Bibliography

Aanderid L, Bakke OM (1985) Tissue distribution of penicillin during constant rate infusion in rats at 71 Ata. Undersea Biomed Res 12: 53–58

Allen MW (1980) Saturation hygiene. Journal of Society of Underwater Technology 6(2): 23–26

Angel A, Halsey MJ, Little H, Meldrum BS, Ross JAS, Rostain JC, Wardley-Smith B (1984) Special effects of drugs at pressure; animal investigations. Philos Trans R Soc Lond B304: 85–93

Ashford MJ, Madonald AG, Wann KT (1984) Hydrostatic pressure modifies the action of octanol and atropine on frog endplate conductance. Br J Pharmacol 83(2): 477–484

Barnard EEP, Elliot DH (1966) Decompression sickness. Paradoxical response to recompression therapy. Br Med J II: 809–810

Bassoe P (1911) Compressed air disease. J Nerve Ment Dis 38: 368–369

Beckman EL, Elliot DH (1974) Dysbarism-related osteonecrosis. U.S. Department of Health, Education and Welfare, Washington

Beeley L (1985) The optimum dose of aspirin as an anti-platelet agent. Br Med J 291: 462

Behnke AR, Yarborough OD (1938) Physiological studies of helium. U.S. Navy Diving Medical Bulletin: 36: 542–548

Bennett PB, Elliot DH (1975) The physiology and medicine of diving. Bailliere Tindall, London

Booth LA (1977) A system for offshore radiology in diving accidents. Radiography 43: 94–96

Bornstein A, Plate E (1911–12) Über chronische Gelenkveränderungen Entstanden durch Press-lufterkrankung. Fortschr Geb Roentgenstrahl 18: 197–206

Boycott AE, Damant GCC, Haldane JS (1908) Prevention of compressed-air illness. J Hyg (Camb) 8: 342–443

Catron PW, Flynn ET (undated) Adjuvant drug therapy for decompression sickness: a review. Naval Medical Research Institute, Bethesda

Cox RAF (1974) The medical examination of commercial divers. Practitioner 212: 861–866

Cox RAF, James PB (1978) Emergency care of diving casualties. Biomedia 1:22

Cox RAF, McIver NKI, King JD, Calder IM (1980) Hypothermia in hyperbaric activities. Lancet II: 1303–1304

Crosbie WA, Clarke MB, Cox RAF, McIver NKI, Anderson IK, Evans HA, Liddle GC, Cowal JL, Brookings CH, Watson DG (1977) Physical characteristics and ventilatory function of 404 commercial divers in the North Sea. Br J Indust Med 34: 19–25

Doran GR, Chaudry L, Brubakk AO, Garrard MP (1985) Hyperbaric liver dysfunction in saturation divers. Undersea Biomed Res 12: 151–164

Dueker CW (1984) Drugs and diving. Undersea J 3: 16–17

Edwards C, Lowry C, Pennefather J (1976) Diving and sub-aquatic medicine. Diving Medical Centre, Sydney

EEC (1979) Directory of information sources for diving operations in Western Europe. Directorate of General and Social Affairs, Luxembourg

EUBS/NPD (1983) Long-term neurological consequences of deep diving

European Diving Technology Committee, Luxembourg Commission of the European Communities (1979) Guidance notes for safe diving, vol 1 and 2. Commission of European Communities, Luxembourg.

Ferris, EB, Engel GL (1952) The clinical nature of high altitude decompression sickness in decompression sickness. In: Fulton JF (ed) Decompression sickness. Saunders, Philadelphia

Futton (1952) Decompression sickness. Saunders, Philadelphia

Golden FStJ, Hervey GR (to be published) Hypothermia ashore and afloat. University Press, Aberdeen

HSE MAI Document (1981). The medical examination of divers. H.M. Stationery Office, London

Keating WR, Hayward MG, McIver NKI (1980) Hypothermia during saturation diving in the North Sea. Br Med J 280: 291

Lancet (1975) Diving doctors. (Editorial) Lancet 1: 440

Linaweaver PG (1977) Physical examination requirements for commercial divers. J Occup Med 19: 817–818.

Mackay DE (1966) Decompression sickness in divers. MD Thesis, Glasgow

Martin RC (1978) The deep sea diver, yesterday, today and tomorrow. Maritime Press, Maryland

Miles S (1962) Underwater medicine. Staples Press, London

Oliver E, Miller JDB, Norman JN (1980) Steroids in secondary drowning. Lancet 1: 105–106

Report to the Lord Commissioners of the Admiralty on Deep Water Diving. HMSO, London (CN/1549 (1907)

Richter R (1975) The medical aspects of drug abuse. Harper and Row, New York

Richter T, Jones C, Nome T, Youngblood DA (1976) The use of drugs and other medical treatment under hyperbaric conditions. Underwater Medical Society, Bethesda

Royal Navy (1980) Diving manual. Ministry of Defence, London

Smith JAR, Norman JN (1979) The use of glucocorticoids in refractory shock. Surg Gynecol Obstet 149: 369–373

Strauss RH (1976) Diving medicine. Grune & Stratton, New York

U.S.Navy (1979) Diving manual. Navy department, Washington

Vallintine R (1981) Divers and diving. Blandford Press, Poole

Walsh JM (1980) Interaction of drugs in the hyperbaric environment. Underwater Medical Society, Bethesda

Werts MF, Shilling CW (1979) Underwater medicine and related sciences: A guide to the literature. Underwater Medical Society, Bethesda

Zinkowski NB (1971) Commercial oilfield diving. Maritime Press, Maryland

Chapter 8

Catering and Hygiene

N. Chalk

> 'Eating is one of life's pleasures — and it outlasts the other!'
> (Brillat-Savarin, 1825, Gourmet and Chef)

In the early days of North Sea exploration, an offshore drilling unit with 50 men aboard was considered a large one, and with the mainland less than 1 h away, food hygiene was treated with a low priority. With the rapid expansion of platforms and flotels in a hostile environment, and a normal population of 500 men or more, the importance of offshore catering and food hygiene has increased beyond the expectations of some of the major oil companies' planners and designers. However, to be fair to them, the difficulties of estimating populations 2 years or so before construction and hook-up are quite considerable. No one could have foreseen the construction problems which have resulted in extended work times and larger work forces. As a result, many platforms have been over-crowded early in their life, with accommodation and catering facilities continually over-stretched, resulting in flooring, catering machinery, and laundry equipment being worn out and broken down before the actual production phase (for which the platform was designed) had commenced its normal routine with the planned population aboard.

The term 'unit' needs definition. This term embraces fixed production platforms, such as the large northern oil platforms and the small southern gas platforms, flotels such as the Aker H3 semisubmersibles, ex-pipe and construction barges modified as accommodation units and the Consafe type of purpose-built flotel, semisubmersible and jack-up drilling units, work barges and all the larger specialist vessels.

In this chapter it is proposed to discuss the catering and food hygiene operations in offshore units and, although most remarks will refer to European activities, the observations and recommendations will also apply to other areas. Obviously in hot climates, far more regard must be paid to food sources, food handling and storage, fly-proofing, double galleys and local habits and customs.

Aboard any units, the catering, cleaning and laundry services are carried out either by independent contract catering companies specialising in this type of work, or by in-house catering companies whose personnel are directly employed by the owner of the vessel concerned (self-catering).

A mixture of other pressures over the past few years has influenced the offshore catering industry, and caused some unease. The offshore catering contractor is often expected to keep up the old image created by the American toolpusher of 'Give 'em a two-inch T-bone for breakfast and don't worry about the cost' attitude, while the shore-side, hard-headed, cost-conscious accountants are closely studying every pared-down quotation from a dozen keen caterers. This gets even more confusing when one caters for vessels whose owners have not been influenced by informal drilling customs, such as traditional European ship-owners with in-built rank structures and attitudes of, 'You old sea cook, cut the cost, you're fiddling anyway'. It is a simple fact that if the caterer cannot make a fair profit, food hygiene aboard will suffer.

Critical Areas

All functions of catering are critical from a hygiene point of view, but it must be remembered that a galley is a workshop, with production deadlines four times a day, 7 days a week. Much danger can be avoided with correct design, and with advice from the user at the early planning stage. One must be realistic however, and accept that most working units have galleys that have been modified, enlarged and altered many times, with a mixture of old and new equipment of varying efficiency (Fig. 8.1).

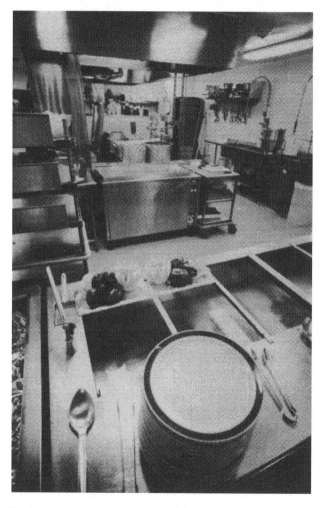

Fig. 8.1.   The galley on a modern production platform.

Food Sources

Most caterers buy supplies from reputable wholesalers, butchers, vegetable mer-
chants and ship's chandlers with much regard for food hygiene, handling and
storage. These suppliers value the bulk business of the offshore industry and rarely
ship poor-quality foodstuffs, but it is a fact that if a caterer is kept to an unworkably
tight budget, he may be tempted to buy cheaply, with subsequent loss of freshness
and quality. Medical officers are advised to inspect caterers' suppliers' premises from
time to time. No good caterer will object. Purchasers should also be aware that
consignments of food, such as meat, can reach offshore installations without tech-
nically being imported and therefore are not subject to normal statutory inspection.

Containers and Transport

Simple steel, unrefrigerated box containers carrying about 4 tons of foodstuffs have
proved to be the most efficient means of moving supplies. They are easily maintained
and can be snatch-lifted by cranes in bad weather. They are simple to clean thoroughly. If a transport delay is expected, they will hold frozen food solid for about 4
days, as long as the container is filled with frozen foods only. Mixed loads hold the
frozen contents solid for proportionately shorter periods. All food containers should
be marked 'FOOD ONLY' and not back-loaded with other goods or garbage.

On arrival aboard the destination unit, food containers should be stored as near to
the final storage point as possible. Food deterioration, including canned goods, is
very rapid if it is stored in damp cartons or sacks.

Stewards unloading containers should wear protective gloves to minimise damage
from the cold. Insensitive fingers carrying cases of frozen meat, heavy cans of
cooking oil, etc. are a sure cause of accidents. Containers must be hoisted by crane
onto the same deck level as the provision stores. Many injuries have been caused by
stewards carrying loads up wet, iron stairs, particularly on moving semisubmersibles
and drill ships.

Storage Offshore

It is obvious that store rooms should be adequate in size, cool, well-ventilated and
clean. The commonest faults in offshore provisions stores, deep freezes and cold
rooms are keeping out-of-date stock and overloading. These faults are more usual on
flotels and seasonal vessels than on platforms. The 'old food' problem is often caused
by the fluctuating work populations. Food is retained on board when the bulk of the
men have left or even when the flotel has been laid up between contracts.

Overloading means stacking goods on the floor nearer and nearer to the door after
the shelves are full. These stacks are often head-high, resulting in the cooks using the
items most accessible, with old stock getting older at the back and the freezer or store
never being cleaned. It should be possible to use up old stock and clean out, but
weather conditions often preclude this and usually there is a contractual necessity to
keep a minimum of 20 days' stock aboard.

Units which have been modified from drilling rigs to accommodation vessels are
most susceptible to this overloading, because the dining room and sleeping quarters
are usually enlarged, but food stores remain as they were when the rig was drilling.

Catering supervisors, medics, and medical officers should periodically check date
marks on food packs, particularly UHT milk, frozen vegetables, eggs and dairy
goods. Frozen meats should be checked for freezer burn and canned meats for
country of origin and the expiry date.

Unfortunately, purpose-built vegetable stores are never provided on any installations. It is estimated that all caterers lose about 10% of their fresh vegetables through poor storage. A cool, dry, well-ventilated, drainable store with grill racking close enough together to discourage high stacking is all that is required.

A good simple guide to food storage offshore can be found in the Code of Practice drawn up by the Institute of Environmental and Offshore Medicine in Aberdeen at the request of the UKOOA Medical Advisory Committee (see, for example, Table 8.1).

Table 8.1. Storage/freezer temperatures[a]

Desired temperature		Storage area
20°C	(70°F)	Galley
5°C	(40°F)	Refrigerator
−6°C	(21°F)	Temporary frozen storage
−18°C	(−0°F) }	Frozen storage offshore
−25°C	(−15°F) }	
−30°C	(−20°F)	Factory cold storage

[a]University of Aberdeen Institute of Environmental and OffshoreMedicine, (1980)

Thawing Frozen Foods

This is one of the most dangerous catering functions, exemplified by a number of deaths in holiday resorts in Britain being attributed to cooked meat soaking up defrosting liquids from thawing poultry on the same work table.

Whenever possible, a separate defrosting area should be set aside and used for nothing else. Where this is not possible, extreme care must be taken in cleaning surfaces, pans, sinks, etc. where defrosting has taken place. Nothing should be artificially defrosted by running water, standing in front of ovens, or thawing on the hot service counter. All meat, fish and poultry should be completely free of frost particles before cooking. The greatest possible care must be taken with large legs of pork and turkeys. At least 24 h natural defrosting at room temperature must be allowed. There are no short cuts to thawing food properly. When microwave ovens are made larger, these concepts will need review. Microwave ovens are often used for smaller items, and of course for reheating. When thawing, it is difficult to ensure that cooks follow the timetable precisely, or even read the chart in the first place. Instruction on use and safety must be positive and frequent. The microwave oven is a useful tool, but must be treated with respect.

Galley Design

First, it must be known how the men are to be fed before proper galley designs can be drawn up. The galley should be thought of as a factory, with raw materials arriving at one end and, after processing, a variety of products emerging from the despatch department at predetermined times. The operator's task is to produce, on time, attractive, tasty, and nutritious food by a variety of methods, without exposing the ingredients to danger from contamination. All poor design, by reducing work efficiency, compresses the time available. When the cook is overworked, for whatever reason, hygiene suffers first. Among the bad habits which will appear, the cook will in his haste not bother to wash his hands when necessary and will wipe perspiration from his face with his apron before cutting cooked meat. Cooks, whose responsibility is underestimated, are entitled to a work place properly designed to smooth their task and positively encourage hygiene.

Floors and Scuppers

The flooring of galleys and ancillary departments should be of light-coloured, dimpled, non-slip, quarry tiles. The 'fall' must be from the centre of the room, be it from actual galley or provisions store, with at least four corner scuppers. Assuming a rectangular galley, it is advisable to build in six scuppers to allow for difficult access to certain drainage points from over-standing machinery or preparation tables. The top traps or gratings should be screwed down to stop workers removing them, and swilling down solid rubbish.

For a cook or galley steward, there is a therapeutic value in the end of shift 'swill down'. The old-fashioned method of cleaning galley floors with plenty of hot, soapy water, vigorously applied with stiff brooms, is still the best way. The regular use of hot water and detergents prevents grease building up, flushes out the scupper system, ensures table and machinery feet are regularly cleaned, and produces an atmosphere encouraging clean surfaces elsewhere. An additional benefit is that a scuppered floor, regularly swilled, discourages floor storage, because if staff need to lift cans, cases and bags before they can clean down, they will find shelf space somewhere.

Galley Bulkheads

Too often, these are painted steel from which the paint easily chips. The resulting chipped-off paint falls onto food preparation surfaces, leaving a scar collecting dirt. Many galleys have stainless steel bulkheads which theoretically are perfect, but aerosol cleaners cannot be used on them. The ideal galley bulkhead is the heavy-duty, plastic-covered sheeting with hard sealed abutments. This lessens echoes, is simply cleaned, and produces less glare. Where the bulkheads meet the floor, a sharp right angle should be avoided. The edge tiles should be curved for easy cleaning. Pot shelves fixed to the bulkhead should not be fitted above head height. Cooks do not wear hard hats in the galley.

Ventilation

The galley should be located so that it can be fitted with opening ports or windows as the galley staff rarely see daylight except on crew changes!

The extraction system must be designed by a ventilation expert, who must take into account the numbers to be fed from the galley, the type and situation of machinery and equipment (i.e. location of roasting ovens, brat pans, baker's oven, grills, etc.). The design engineers must allow for concentrated extraction from steam and fume locations, and general air changes in other areas of the galley. When extraction is too powerful, food gets cold quickly.

Food Handlers' Toilet Facilities

Close to, but not adjoining the galley, there should be a urinal, W.C. and hand-wash facilities solely for the use of food handlers. The W.C. should have a pedal-operated flush, and the wash basin should have elbow taps with an air hand dryer nearby. A mirror should not be provided, so that food handlers will not be tempted to comb their hair or squeeze facial pustules after washing their hands. 'NOW WASH YOUR HANDS' notices must be very evident. Extractor fans are essential.

Preparation Surfaces

The normal lipped, heavy-gauge stainless steel work top is excellent. The only disadvantage from a cook's point of view is that chopping boards must always be used (polypropylene, *not* wooden boards). Heavily scarred and scratched surfaces should be replaced.

The fewer drawers fitted in these work tables the better, as drawers usually become repositories for anything without a proper home, including piping tubes, apple cores, and old finger bandages.

Catering Machinery (Galley)

Depending on the production capacity, most of the following items of equipment are required: roasting ovens, baking-confectioner's ovens, steam ovens, dough prover, bain-marie, deep fryers, salamanders, potato peeling machine, potato chipping machine, mixers (with shred, slice and mince attachments), slicing machines, griddles, boiling plates, refrigerators, waste disposers, pastry rollers, brat pans, lowerators and serving counter.

Though the machinery and equipment in a galley is very expensive, it generally pays to buy top-quality items in the long term. It is better buy as many items from the one manufacturer as possible. This ensures uniform height, fixing, spares systems, accessibility, replacement, and cleaning procedures, and saves money. There are many old-established reputable manufacturers in Europe who have their own foundry. The easier a machine is to clean, the more often it gets cleaned. The problems of siting machinery may be compared with placing furniture in one's own sitting room — everyone thinks it would be better in a different position. In the galley, the siting is also dictated to some extent by main bulkheads, doors, windows, and of course the serving counter. The galley's sub-departments (bakery area, pan wash, vegetable preparation, defrosting area, service) solve half the location problem by their requirement for specialised machinery.

Assuming that the galley is for more than 100 men, the roasting ovens, fryers, boiling plates, brat pans, steamers and griddles should form a back-to-back island in the centre of the main galley, with an extractor hood over the whole group.

The most important hygiene difficulty arises in ensuring reasonable access for maintenance and repair, whilst sealing off spaces to prevent the accumulation of grease and spillage down the back and sides, which also causes a fire hazard. The provision of all machinery from the same manufacturer usually overcomes this, as it will have interconnecting stainless steel spaces and kickplates. This problem is also helped by allowing small, stainless steel work surfaces between, for example, fryers and griddle, brat pan and boiling plate.

Handles and switches on ovens, mixers and grills constitute dangerous dirt traps.

By their very nature they are difficult to clean, switches being knurled to allow grip, and a cook has to operate switches with greasy fingers. All electrical switches must be cleaned carefully, and all loose handles should be tightened for safety.

Cleaning of Specific Items

Ovens

Regular cleaning of the insides of ovens presents difficulties. Most proprietary brands of oven cleaners are required to be left for some time before cleaning, and most ovens on offshore installations are in continuous use. An apparently dirty oven inside rarely presents a health hazard, as the continuous high working temperatures will kill most bacteria.

Potato Chipping Machine

This should be scrubbed with hot, soapy water and rinsed with cold. The chessboard cutter should be removed periodically and boiled in a pan not used for food. Slides and return spring need re-greasing occasionally. Inspect by looking underneath the drop hole.

Potato Peeling Machine

Scrub with hot, soapy water. It is vital to ensure that the free-flow waste pipe is clear; frequent running, unloaded, with flowing water keeps pipe and drain clear.

Griddle

The cooking surface should be scraped while hot and then rubbed with a proprietary volcanic block to remove finer burnt debris. The grease drain can be cleaned with a teapot brush on a wire. The top surface should be oiled immediately after cleaning to prevent rust.

Boiling Plates

Clean in the same way as the griddle.

Deep Fryers

Oil should be drained as necessary. It is pointless to drain daily, as this froths the oil and reduces its viscosity. No bacteria can live in frying oil in daily use, as the cooking temperature is above 400°F and it rarely cools below 200°F. After every use, however, top lips and edges of the inside of the pan should be wiped with a dry cloth. Wiping inside with a wet cloth is dangerous, as squeezed water will trickle into the oil and, when the fryer is switched to full heat, will cause the oil to foam, rise rapidly and spill over the top. This is the cause of many kitchen fires. Happily all fryers are now fitted with thermostats, but years ago cooks would spit into hot fat — if it spat back the fat was hot enough!

Bain-Marie

Traditionally 'Mary's bath' is a tank containing hot water in which to stand containers of liquid to keep them hot. If pots of soup, sauce, or custard were kept on a boiling plate the contents would burn on the bottom. Modern bains-marie are of two types, either continuously heated water in a recessed tank, or a dry, heated space set in a serving counter. The water bain-marie is preferable for efficiency and cleaning, but does cause dangerous swill-out problems in a ship or moveable unit in rough seas. A service counter with hot water under the serving trays, swilling from one tray of food to another and over the server's feet, may be Chaplinesque, but is very annoying. Hygienically, the danger is the natural reluctance of catering staff to drain and clean out the bains-marie after every service. The previous day's menu is often apparent from the bits of food floating in the bains-marie. Continual clearing is essential, as the water does not boil. If neglected, the food junk is a perfect environment for breeding bacteria. Disinfectant should never be used.

Serving Counter

Most of the points concerning hygiene are covered in the previous paragraph, because usually the bain-marie and serving counter are one integral unit. The serving counter must, of course, be constructed of stainless steel with well-fitting inserts, lids and doors. The doors should be removed weekly and the lower running slides cleaned thoroughly. The inspecting medical officer must kneel to look at the back of the hot cupboard space for forgotten foodstuffs pushed to the back. The whole should be washed with clean water and mild detergent then, when dry, polished with a dry cloth.

Ice-Cream Dispensers

Most units nowadays have at least one soft ice-cream dispensing machine. These machines are extremely difficult to keep bacteriologically clean. Pathogenic bacteria can almost always be cultured from them and they are a health hazard if not thoroughly cleaned more often than the maker's recommendations. Clear, positive instructions to the camp boss or chief cook should include a hard and fast rule that *all* removable parts — filters, taps, and detachable drums — should be removed from the machine and boiled in salt water three times in every 24 h. Two complete sets should be kept in use; one on the machine and the other boiled and put in sealed, clear plastic bags in the camp boss's office or chief-cook's desk.

Dining Room

Dining rooms offshore vary in standard from cheap, clattering, harsh workmen's canteens to softly lit, carpeted first-class restaurants. Whatever the appearance, all standards must be acceptable from the point of view of food hygiene.

Where a unit is of old design, not permitting a 'boots and overalls off' discipline, and where drilling involves oil-based mud, the basic plastic, easily scrubbable floors, chairs, tables and bulkheads are best. At the other end of the scale, where no drilling takes place and accommodation areas are only entered in house clothing, then as much comfort as possible in an otherwise harsh environment is to be advocated. It is well known that during the often lengthy construction phase the riggers, welders, scaffolders, and other heavy workers are called 'bears', but it is my experience that given the opportunity to live in a civilised manner, the great majority of them respond well. There will always be the few who get into bed wearing their boots and overalls, but if the remainder know that rules are for everyone's benefit, and those rules of behaviour are instigated from the very beginning, life becomes more civilised for all concerned. To be specific about dining room cleaning and management is merely to highlight common sense. Quite simply, everything must be cleaned thoroughly after every meal. When large numbers are to be fed, beverage and cold drink points should not be at the end of the service counter. This causes bottlenecks at peak periods when the queue must be kept moving. Fresh fruit, bread, cheese-boards, etc. should also be in the main body of the dining room, to prevent the end-of-service-counter traffic causing congestion. Some designers blindly follow the example of onshore cafeterias where all items on offer are in a straight line, not realising that this is for the benefit of the check-out cashier. This is not required offshore.

Hard floors must be mopped with frequent changes of hot, soapy water immediately after every meal. Unit offshore installation managers must cooperate with the caterers to allow the dining room to be closed for sufficient time for thorough cleaning, and floors and tables to dry properly. Depending on traffic, floors should be thoroughly scrubbed, preferably by machine, at least once per week. This is best done after the midnight meal and before breakfast. If floors are polished, care must be taken always to use a non-slip polish.

For a dining room in heavy use, the best chairs are those of one-piece, heavy moulded plastic, which are of Scandinavian design. These are easily cleaned, whereas dimpled plastic or upholstered chairs always look grubby. Table tops must be of stain-proof, heavy-duty plastic laminate. Many people offshore don't bother to use a side plate, and consequently knife scores on tables rapidly become difficult to clean properly and table tops start to chip. Drink and ice-cream dispensers must be dismantled and cleaned daily. The dangers of an unhygienic ice-cream machine are obvious. Butter should be portion-wrapped and all sauce bottles should be wiped clean regularly. The practice of the caterer buying bulk sauces and continually topping up old sauce bottles should be vigorously discouraged. The problem of a dirty plate collection point and plate scrape bins is a difficult one to solve. To enjoy a meal and then gaze into a bucket of other people's leftovers is aesthetically offensive, while swing-lid bins are not the whole answer as the lids usually get messy very quickly. Specially designed stainless steel trolleys are now available.

The plate-wash room must be separate from the galley pan-wash tanks, and preferably a separate room allowing for good plate storage. All chipped plates and crockery must be discarded immediately. The plate-wash machine must be of the largest capacity and power acceptable by the unit and spare parts must be in stock at all times.

The cold buffet is often on display in the dining room. This usually consists of a large variety of cold meats, fish, salads and hors d'oeuvres, which is laid out on a table or cold counter and is completely open. It is advisable to provide a refrigerated display cabinet with glass sneeze screen. Meal times are often protracted offshore, and the buffet items could well be exposed to a warm atmosphere for 3 h. After meals, all items must be removed from their tray or container and doubtful and edge-curled foodstuffs thrown away, while good food should be refrigerated immediately. No cooked meats should be put out on display more than twice. Tinned fish should not be displayed in its original can. In warm weather it is better to put out cold foods little and often throughout the meal times. The display is not so impressive, but then it is much fresher and so much safer.

The cutlery dispensing trays should be of the clean, plastic, horizontal type. The containers in which the cutlery stands upright are unhygienic because the cutlery becomes inverted, ensuring that spoon bowls, fork tines and knife blades are fingered by everyone else during their selection. The horizontal containers allow easy visual identification.

Cooks' Tools

Great advances have been made in the last few years in the design and manufacture of cooks' knives, carving forks and cutting boards. Although efficient from a functional point of view, the traditional cook's knife with integral blade and tang and riveted handled sides was a hygienic disaster. The rivets became loose, allowing dirt to accumulate between the tang and the handle's sides and contaminate the cook's hands. Modern knives with moulded polypropylene handles are the only knives which should be allowed in galleys. Where possible, all tools should go through the plate-washing machine, as these machines usually project the hottest water on board.

Wooden chopping boards are more comfortable for a cook to use, but harbour bacteria in the inevitable scars. Polypropylene cutting boards must be used. An often unnoticed danger spot, regrettably forgotten by many cooks, is the wheel and blade on the underpart of the rotary can-opener handle. This becomes gummed up with fruit juice, rust, and meat fat, and this old accumulation then drops into the can being opened. A daily clean with scrubbing brush and hot, soapy water is all that is required.

Food Handlers

It is necessary to emphasise the necessity for food handlers to have short hair, short fingernails, regular bathing habits and clean, white clothing. Their cleanliness should be regularly inspected and those with septic spots, runny ears, open sneezing or infected fingers rejected. There are other small points which may not be obvious, but must be borne in mind.

All cooks know that smoking where food is stored, prepared or served is not allowed, but very few know why. They should be told that the smoke or ash is not in the least harmful to foodstuffs, unsightly as it may be. The danger is mucus from lips and mouths spreading bacteria by coming into contact with food. The simplest example of this is when a food handler removes a cigarette from his mouth, carefully rests it, hot end out, on the side of the bread tray or edge of a table. The moisture from the mouth is then transmitted to a surface in contact with food, and this mucus is also on his fingers.

It is difficult to enforce the wearing of disposable hats by cooks and food handlers, but every effort must be made. Apart from hair falling into food, a hat discourages unconscious head scratching. Cooks boning out meat should always wear a chain mail glove on the non-cutting hand, and if practicable, a chain mail short apron.

Food handlers should be encouraged to wash their hands frequently, not just after using a lavatory, which is essential, but after opening boxes of meat, handling boxes of vegetables or any package which could have been floor-stored or dirty. Regular FFI inspections must be strictly enforced and recorded.

Nutrition Offshore

How does one recommend a nutritious, balanced diet to several hundred hungry men, from sophisticated managers and engineers to husky scaffolders, riggers and roustabouts who are on the move in the open air for 12 h at a time? The answer is to give them what they want, which is a lot of meat and piles of chipped potatoes, balanced with as large a variety of vegetables, salads, fruit and wholemeal bread as is convenient and practicable.

If a perfectly balanced bill of fare is provided, men will complain. One can only ensure that a diet rich in vitamins and fibre, including polyunsaturated fats, is available for those who want it. To a shore-based observer, the bulk intake of the heavy manual worker offshore is enormous. The last calculation of all food usage over a 1-month winter period (1979–1980) resulted in a man day consumption of 4.6 kg (10 lb 3 oz), excluding beverage liquid. Of this, 0.94 kg (2 lb 1½ oz) was meat products, that is, whole meat (roasts, chops, cold cuts, etc.), bacon, sausage, poultry and mince. This consumption was during the construction and hook-up phase of a large northern platform in winter and so was probably a near-maximum figure.

It is noticeable, however, that over the last few years, more men are avoiding fried potato dishes, puddings and cakes. Salad consumption has doubled in 5 years, and more people ask for polyunsaturated margarine and wholemeal bread. It is worth remarking that this trend is mainly among the younger workers. Every effort should be made by management to educate men into at least thinking about the dangers of obesity and so avoiding it, because it is a growing problem offshore. Alternative menus providing fewer calories and more fibre should be provided at every meal.

Routine Health and Hygiene Inspections

Weekly hygiene inspections should be performed by the offshore medics, who should submit a brief written report to the installation manager. More formal medical and hygiene inspections of all offshore installations should be carried out about every 6 months. These inspections should be conducted by either a physician or one of his nursing staff. Nurses often have a better eye for matters of hygiene than doctors, and with the increasing employment of women offshore there is a strong argument for these routine inspections being conducted fairly regularly by members of the nursing staff.

On installations where standards appear to be inadequate or where there are threats to hygiene, such as temporary over-crowding, it may be necessary to carry out inspections at more frequent intervals than 6 monthly. The results of each inspection should be carefully documented, and it is helpful if they are conducted to a standard format (e.g. that recommended by the UKOOA which is given in Appendix 7).

The following notes are offered for the guidance of nurses or physicians carrying out these inspections.

Cabins

Note cleanliness, tidiness, evidence of over-crowding and the state of the beds and linen.

Toilets

The toilets used by the catering staff must have a notice stating 'NOW WASH YOUR HANDS' to comply with food and hygiene regulations. In all toilets note the cleanliness, proper functioning, maintenance, provision of adequate toilet paper, whether the doors lock, the state of ventilation, etc.

Washrooms

Note cleanliness, whether there are broken basins, whether the faucets are operating properly, and the provision of soap, towels, etc. Also note whether a tub (either fixed or collapsible) is available for the treatment of cases of hypothermia.

Mess Room

Notice the cleanliness, tidiness, ventilation, lighting and any evidence of over-crowding.

Laundry Room

Note the cleanliness, tidiness, type of laundering being done, whether the machinery is in a good state of repair, and the condition of the walls and floors. Particularly note whether ventilation is adequate.

First-Aid Room/Sick Bay

Note the size, the adequacy of lighting and ventilation, noise levels, how many beds and whether any of them are used by the medic for sleeping, the working areas available, the provision of essential furniture, such as examination couches, cup-boards, refrigerator, steriliser, etc. Note also the proximity and condition of the toilets associated with the sick bay, what showers and washing facilities are available, and the general cleanliness and tidiness of the room. Also note what telephone communications exist between the first-aid room and the rest of the rig.

The Medic

The name of the medic and his qualifications should be noted along with the name of his alternate and his qualifications. Comment upon his training, what refresher courses he has been on and how long he has been on the installation; any impressions that you may have gained regarding his competence and standing with the rest of the crew are valuable. Also make a note of his normal work routine and whether it involves other duties apart from medical, such as hygiene surveillance, first-aid instruction, general clerical duties, etc. It is also important to document your comments on the keeping of proper medical records and the Controlled Drugs Register.

Drugs and Dressings

Comments should be made on the adequacy of the stocks and whether they comply with the current regulations, whether any drugs are out of date, whether the containers are adequately labelled and whether there is any evidence of unusual consumption or use of drugs. At the same time, the general state of tidiness of the drug cupboards should be noted and also whether the stretchers, resuscitators, sterilisers, etc. are in working order and properly maintained.

Food and Drink Dispensers

These should be carefully examined, noting the types and the frequency with which they are maintained and cleaned.

Galley

Note the cleanliness, tidiness, washing facilities available for the staff (which should be separate from the food preparation area), and whether there are soap and nail brushes provided. Also note the condition of any towels used for drying crockery, and whether the faucets are operating properly. Comment upon the general repair and maintenance of the galley area, and note whether there is any unusual accumulation of grease or dirt, especially around extractor hoods. Notice should be taken of the adequacy of the lighting, the condition of the floors, and enquiry made about the frequency and procedure of the routine chemical and bacteriological analysis of the drinking water.

Stores

Note whether they are tidy and clean, whether there is food on the floor, or if there is any damaged or out-dated food. Comment should also be made if there is evidence of an excess of food. Lighting and ventilation should be inspected, with particular observation kept for evidence of infestation with cockroaches or mice. Note whether any food is being stored without a cover.

Cold Stores

Note the temperature of the cold store and the cleanliness, tidiness and condition of the food stored in it. Note whether the cold stored is used only for perishable food or whether other goods are stored there also. Note whether the food is used on a rotation principle, the oldest being consumed first, and whether the cold store safety alarm is working.

Vegetable Store

Note should be made of the location and size of the vegetable store and whether it is used for other purposes. Comment on the condition of its contents and whether garbage is stored in the same area.

Garbage

Note how much garbage is about, how it is stored, how it is disposed of and whether there is any smell from the garbage areas.

Recreation Room

Note the general state of cleanliness, tidiness, whether the furniture is in a good state of repair or whether it is excessively worn, the decorative state of the room, the working condition of the television or other equipment and whether there is an adequate supply of books, games and other recreational facilities.

Food Preparation and Serving

Note should be taken of the choice of food, whether fresh fruit and vegetables are available, the quality of the food and whether it is attractively presented, whether the crew are satisfied with the catering or whether they have complaints. Enquiries should be made regarding the utilisation of leftover food, whether a lot of food is re-heated or left out for long periods and on what criteria decisions are taken to dispose of unused food.

Catering Personnel

Note the number of catering personnel, including cabin stewards, their general appearance and cleanliness, paying particular attention to their hair and fingernails and whether they have evidence of open wounds, sores or sepsis, or discharging ears. Note any unhygienic habits they may have, and whether any have had recent illnesses. Note also whether adequate protective clothing is worn and whether they have their heads covered when working in the galley. Note should be made of the dates of their last medical examinations and where and by whom they were performed.

Testing of Potable Water

The potable water should be examined chemically and bacteriologically at regular intervals. If the unit is making its own water, by distillation, an examination every 3 months is adequate. If, however, the installation is receiving bunkered water from supply vessels, examination should be carried out at least every month, as contamination from bunkered water is common. The samples of water should be taken by the medic, as one of his regular duties, into sterile containers and with careful flaming of faucets before collecting the aliquot. The samples should then be despatched to the laboratory for analysis as quickly as possible. The examinations are usually performed by the local public analyst or public health laboratory.

Bibliography

Aston G, Tiffney J (1977) A guide to improving food hygiene. Initial ideas. Saunders, Philadelphia
Mottram VH, Arnold E (1979) Human nutrition. Arnold, London
University of Aberdeen Institute of Environmental and Offshore Medicine (1980) Environmental health
   — offshore installations. The University, Aberdeen

Chapter 9

Dental Problems Offshore

D.J.G. Pyper

With the exception of trauma and accidents, the majority of dental problems may be prevented, providing each person has had routine dental inspections. There are no specific problems which arise offshore, but because of the environment and the lack of on-site professional help, a simple dental lesion may become acute. At present, a dental emergency which cannot be simply treated is sent ashore. This is not only costly, but causes a manpower shortage due to the long delay often experienced in obtaining dental treatment.

The majority of employees in the offshore industry are young and fit. The commonest dental problems are: (a) dental decay and the result of its treatment; and (b) periodontal disease (pyorrhoea and its sequelae).

It is obvious that prevention of dental problems is far more important than treating established disease. Examining GPs are best placed to assess the employee's oral health at the time of the routine pre-employment examination. No company yet insists upon a separate dental examination as part of that initial medical check-up, but oral health is an important part of a person's general health.

Ideally, a dental examination should be carried out at the same time as the medical examination. As few dentists work in the same clinics as their medical colleagues, a compromise is necessary, and for this reason it is advocated that the physician should carry out a simple dental examination when conducting the medical examination. The dental light can be replaced by an adjustable light which provides excellent illumination of the mouth; the dental chair is replaced by an examination couch. The only additional instrument required is a simple mouth mirror.

Questions which can be asked of the employee to make the doctor's job easier are:

1. Have you a regular dentist?
2. When was your last visit to a dentist?
3. Do you have toothache?
4. Do your teeth ache after eating and drinking?
5. Do your gums bleed after brushing?
6. Do you wear false teeth?
7. Have you ever had your teeth X-rayed?

If a full clinical dental examination by a dental surgeon is required, it will include an examination of the teeth, soft tissues and an external examination of the face and lips, including the temporomandibular joint and its associated muscles. A medical history will be reviewed and routine X-rays taken to show teeth and underlying bone in order to reveal any pathological problems which may be hidden from a clinical examination. Once all this information is correlated the dental surgeon can then give an opinion as to whether the employee is fit to proceed offshore.

Dental Standards

The minimum standards of dental health acceptable for those working offshore must ensure that the employee is free of any disability which may prevent him from continuing his offshore work. The dentist must, therefore, determine that he is: (a) pain-free, (b) infection-free, both periodontal and dental; and (c) has the optimum function and comfort from his teeth.

In the offshore situation there is no local dentist available to deal with the employee's problems and in many cases evacuated personnel must return to their home bases, perhaps hundreds of miles from the nearest shore base, to obtain treatment. The introduction of shorter periods offshore has meant that employees can benefit from regular dental treatment planned during their shore leaves. This should mean that, with the exception of trauma cases, there should be less need for evacuation for dental problems.

After clinical examination such as that described the dentist will decide that the patient is in one of the following categories:

1. Able to proceed offshore with no treatment required
2. Able to proceed offshore, but will require treatment soon (during shore leave)
3. Only able to proceed offshore after emergency treatment has been carried out, e.g. extractions or root canal therapy
4. Unable to proceed offshore until extensive dental treatment has been completed (cases most at risk)

Category 2 does not include dental extractions. A person who has had a tooth extracted should stay ashore for at least 3 days in case problems such as haemorrhage or infection should occur and these can be treated. Extractions should, therefore, be carried out at the beginning of shore leave, not the end.

Dental Jurisprudence

There are some problems in providing dental services offshore, related to the Dentists Act 1984. Under Section 38 of the Act, it is unlawful for anyone to give or even to suggest that he is prepared to give, any treatment or advice, including treatment or advice in connection with the fitting, insertion or fixing of dentures, artificial teeth or other dental appliances such as is normally given by a dentist *unless* he is registered in the Dentists Register or Medical Register, or is an enrolled dental hygienist or dental therapist practising dentistry under the Ancillary Dental Workers Regulations. A dentist who knowingly or through neglect of this duty enables a person to do dental work which that person is not permitted by law to do, is liable to proceedings for misconduct.

It is unethical for a dental practitioner to delegate to a person who is neither a registered dental practitioner nor an enrolled auxiliary, responsibility for instructing patients in the principles and practice of oral hygiene unless:

1. The dentist is satisfied that the person to whom the responsibility is delegated is fully competent to discharge it.

2. The practitioner understands that he is personally responsible for whatever instruction is given in his name.

It is apparent from this that both dentists and medics may face a dilemma regarding dental treatment offshore.

The Dentists Act was passed to protect the public and the dentists. It was not passed to prevent people from receiving care and attention in dental emergencies wherever they may occur.

Dental First Aid

The provision of good dental care offshore relies on good secondary diagnosis by the medic, who must be able to get as much information as possible about the patient's signs and symptoms and relay them to the dentist ashore so that a reasonable diagnosis can be made over the telephone and emergency first-aid treatment prescribed.

It is important that medics be acquainted with dental matters and are able to recognise common dental problems so that clinical descriptions can be given accurately to those ashore. This instruction must be given either in the form of formal training or on a separate course over a short period, as medics have no formal dental training in their SRN nursing course. Most service-trained medics are given a short dental course in their training periods with the military services and are therefore in an enviable position to recognise true dental emergencies when they occur. They are also able to communicate better with the dentist or doctor ashore to provide treatment and organise the care of the employee.

The medic must, therefore, be able to recognise causes of toothache, swellings in and around the mouth, and various facial pains, and to provide emergency treatment for trauma cases. He must also be able to communicate his clinical findings to a dentist ashore. The SRN training of the medic rarely includes much time on dental matters, which are usually only covered in a cursory manner. However, it is important that at least a working knowledge be gained during his training. This could be learned in the casualty department of a hospital or by spending some time with a dental surgeon who is acquainted with the offshore industry. Formal training will eventually be required by the Offshore Installations and Pipeline Works (First-Aid) Regulations.

Most routine dental cases presenting offshore may be treated with analgesics or antibiotics under the direction of a dentist or medical adviser and the patient can then be sent ashore for routine treatment either on the next available helicopter or on his next leave. The difficult problems arise when the emergency occurs in conditions which make evacuation impossible, in which case the medics may well be called upon to provide more than just analgesic or antibiotic therapy.

Among the medical equipment carried should be an emergency dental kit similar to those used on board Her Majesty' ships. The kit should be simple and basic in content so that after formal training qualified medical attendants can use it in an emergency. This kit should contain:

Pen torch
Mouth mirror
Probe
Excavators
Plastic instruments
Scissors
Spatula
Forceps
Irrigating syringe
Cotton wool
Gauze squares
Mixing slab
Temporary dressings, e.g. Cavit, Septodont products
Dental bib
Mouth prop
Chip syringe

The commonest presenting symptom of non-traumatic origin is toothache. This may be acute or chronic and vary in severity and the commonest cause of toothache is an inflammation of the pulp of the tooth (pulpitis). Other causes may be cracked or leaking fillings, a fractured tooth or sensitive cementum. Mild analgesics will usually calm the painful tooth and control the pain. However, it may be necessary to consult with the doctor or dentist ashore if more potent drugs are to be prescribed, e.g. dextropropoxyphene or dihydrocodeine, both of which have side effects and prolonged administration should be avoided.

In cases where the patient has lost a filling or broken part of a tooth and cannot be evacuated for dental treatment ashore, a temporary dressing can be inserted to relieve symptoms. This can be done by isolating the tooth with cotton wool rolls, drying it with cotton buds or the air chip syringe and inserting the dressing with a plastic instrument. With the introduction of ready-mixed dressing materials such as Cavit or gutta-percha, the insertion of temporary dressings has become fairly simple. However, the old-fashioned dressing of oil of cloves mixed with zinc oxide powder is still very popular because of the soothing effect of the clove oil.

Crowns may become dislodged and loose following minor trauma. Re-cementing of the crown with chewing gum, tissue paper, glue and various other non-dental products has been successful, but it is easier and less irritating to the tooth and the tissues surrounding the tooth if a medic prepares a creamy mix of dental cement such as Kalzinol (a zinc oxide–oil of cloves preparation) and re-cements the crown.

The true dental abscess, which is the result of pulpitis, may well be confused with a periodontal gum abscess caused through localised periodontal disease. Antibiotic therapy will usually relieve symptoms without the use of an analgesic. The prescription of the antibiotic can only be given under the direction of the doctor or dentist ashore. A mouth wash should also be used. An excellent mouth wash for this is chlorhexidine, although prolonged use of it will stain the teeth and surrounding tissues.

It must be emphasised that medics should not attempt to carry out any treatment, except for the relief of symptoms, and then only under the doctor or dentist's directions. Not only may this be illegal, but it may complicate follow-up treatment in the dental surgery ashore. A letter should always accompany the employee once he has been evacuated to the shore dentist with an outline of the signs and symptoms and the treatment carried out.

No emergency dental kit should be without a denture repair kit. This may be one of the new dental adhesive cements — the cyano acrylic adhesives — or the normal acrylic denture repair kit which is easily available from dental suppliers.

Dental Problems in Diving

Diving is now a highly specialised professional occupation, requiring elaborate back-up facilities and specialist medical and dental advice. The introduction of saturation diving has brought its own dental problems. Previously, the only problem was ensuring that the diver could form a seal round his mouthpiece and whether he had sufficient teeth left in his mouth to bite on the flanges of the mouthpiece to keep it stable. Miles' (1962) only reference to dentistry in *Underwater Medicine* is, 'dentures should be removed before diving'. But this simple instruction produces problems for those divers with edentulous mouths. Without teeth they have great difficulty in retaining the mouthpiece. Specialist flanges have been individually made to give greater retention to the mouthpiece and help with forming an adequate seal. Unfortunately, these are expensive and alternative methods have had to be devised.

The solution to many of these problems has been the use of the full face mask and surface demand gas supplies. The wearing of loose removable dentures or appliances while diving is dangerous, as they may become dislodged and cause respiratory obstruction, especially in the event of unconsciousness.

Few dental problems occur in divers who have well-kept mouths, but mouths with many restorations are more likely to cause problems. The emphasis is on the prevention of dental disease in this specialist group of employees. In saturation diving it is impossible to carry out routine treatments. Even the relief of pain with analgesics proves difficult, and the diver must wait to be decompressed before treatment can be satisfactorily concluded.

It is recommended that the commercial divers, and especially saturation divers, should have a detailed examination of their teeth at the time of their annual medical examinations. The saturation diver is more at risk from the fact that treatment may be very difficult during an extended hyperbaric exposure.

If the diver attends his own dentist it is important that he informs him that he does dive commercially and that he is working in a hyperbaric environment. Sensitive teeth and broken fillings should be treated and repaired before diving to minimise the likelihood of problems under pressure. Often patients have sensitivity around the necks of their teeth caused by recession of the gum margins exposing cementum and root areas. Changes in temperature can cause pain in these areas. Cold gases breathed by the diver are likely to be a major cause of this kind of discomfort. The use of one of the specialised toothpastes such as Sensodyne is recommended for this, using the toothpaste as a cream applied to the sensitive area.

Full upper and lower dentures must not be worn whilst diving as they can easily become dislodged and impact in the pharynx with fatal consequences. Partial dentures may be worn if they are clasped firmly to the remaining teeth and are retentive so they cannot be dislodged.

The flange on the mouthpiece must be capable of forming a positive seal. The 'rubber stops' on the flange should only provide additional retention by biting in case the mouthpiece becomes dislodged. Divers who continually bite onto these stops complain of temporomandibular joint discomfort after dives. This discomfort is usually only of a temporary nature, but should it persist for long periods and cause distress, then consultation with a doctor or dentist for treatment of the temporomandibular joint syndrome should be sought.

The problem of barodontalgia has been well documented in a paper by Carlson et al. (1983). They suggest that 'dental pain is of two types, dull and non-localised, or sharp and well-defined'. Their recommendations for treatment are:

1.   Sharp localised pain may be eliminated by removing the restorations and applying a liner to seal the dentine tubules prior to placement of the restoration.
2.   Dull non-localised pain suggests the need to evaluate for endodontic therapy.

Their paper establishes a possible cause for the discomfort experienced by some divers, but it is the writer's experience that the problems mainly arise from inadequate restorations. Routine, double-lining of cavities has proved successful in these patients.

Dental Treatment

The Diver and the Dentist

A dentist faced with a diving patient has a responsibility to ensure the diver is dentally fit to dive. That is, the diver's mouth is infection-free and he is aware of any potential problems in the mouth. Large restorations in teeth should be checked for soundness and vitality. Acute or chronic pulpitis is difficult to treat in a hyperbaric situation and may well lead to further problems for the diver if he cannot concentrate on his job because of the discomfort of toothache.

Buried teeth do not usually cause problems, but if there is a risk of partial impaction or acute infection removal is justified, for the safety of the diver.

X-rays should be routinely taken to ensure that small cavities can be treated early to prevent symptoms. Double-linings will ensure that exposed dentine tubules are protected from exposure to the oral cavity or thermal change. Non-vital teeth must be investigated and endodontic therapy undertaken. The canals should be sealed before diving as a partially completed canal may not remain symptomless in the hyperbaric environment.

Divers should not dive with dentures unless these are secured to crowns or natural teeth that will prevent them becoming dislodged. They should be able to form a seal without dentures in their mouths.

The Medic

The successful resolution of a dental problem occurring in a patient under pressure will depend upon the medic obtaining a detailed description of the signs and symptoms and communicating these to the doctor or dentist. The further management of the patient and the dive will depend upon the presumed diagnosis.

The diver under routine treatment by his dentist will have informed him of his occupation so that extensive treatment will not be undertaken before a dive. The medic will usually be dealing with trauma, cracked teeth or fillings or infections.

He can do little for the diver in a saturation chamber with a cracked filling or broken tooth, except use mild analgesics or allow the diver to repair the tooth temporarily with one of the simple dental dressings on the market, e.g. Septodont products or Cavit. These can be passed through the medical hatch and the diver instructed how to apply the dressing. Pain from a cracked tooth or filling is due to the exposure of sensitive dentine. Desensitising pastes or liquids may be used as a temporary measure and extremely hot or cold food and drink should be avoided.

If the diver has an acute abscess he will be feverish and unwell. He must not be allowed to continue working. The patient is likely to have a raised pulse and fever, and a swelling in association with the abscess. He will require analgesics, antibiotics and referral to a dental surgeon as soon as he surfaces.

Bibliography

Carlson OG, Halverson BA, Triplett RG (1983) Dentin permeability under hyperbaric conditions as a possible cause of barodontalgia. Undersea Biomed Res 10: 23–28
Cooper R (1976) Dental problems in medical practice. Heinemann, London
Crabb HSM (1969) Emergency dental treatment. Wright, Bristol
Mack PJ, Hobson RS, Astell J (1985) Dental factors in scuba mouthpiece design. Br Dent J: 141–142
Miles S (1962) Underwater medicine. Staples Press, London

Chapter 10

Investigation of Fatal and Non-Fatal Accidents

I.M. Calder

The full, detailed and objective investigation of any accident is essential for three reasons:

1. To establish the facts of the case to dispel suspicion and speculation
2. To enable changes in procedure and equipment to be made to prevent a future recurrence
3. To establish the cause of the accident with accuracy so that proper and appropriate compensation can be determined

Although attention focuses on the *fatal* accident, a unified appraisal must be made of all accidents. In the case of the fatal accident it is usually mandatory that at some time the local legal authorities are involved, and this may also be so where injuries are *non*-fatal. It has been suggested by Goad (1981) that non-punitive recording of 'near-miss' accidents should be made, especially in diving incidents. Autopsies should be performed following *all* fatal accidents. Even following a major disaster where there may appear to be a common cause of death, proper autopsies will establish a pattern of injury, which will be a vital piece of information in explaining the disaster and evaluating the efficiency of the rescue and escape procedures. This was emphasised by R. D. Menzies (1979, personal communication), who performed some 638 autopsies following a major disaster.

The Fatal Accident

Legal Investigative Aspects

The only responsibility of the medical practitioner is to certify the fact of death. To endeavour to give a cause of death without full investigation enters the realm of speculation which is inaccurate and can be dangerous.

Once the fact of death is established there is usually a due process of law to be followed. Systems of medico-legal investigation of sudden, violent or unexplained death fall into three main groups, which have developed as a result of different historical backgrounds. Countries with a common law background, which include England and many of its colonies, ex-colonies and dominions, have adopted the coroner system.

In Scotland a similar system is operated through the procurator fiscal. In some states of North America radical reform is being carried out with the loss of some advantages of the coroner system. Under the medical examiner system of the United States, a medically qualified executive officer is appointed with greatly reduced powers and often a lack of legal knowledge compared with the English coroner.

In Norway following a fatal accident the local police initiate the investigation. If a medical practitioner cannot certify a cause of death from knowledge of the circumstances and from the external examination of the body, an autopsy is arranged if possible. However, in the case of an industrial accident (which includes diving), the body has to be transported to a suitable centre.

Further specialist investigation is carried out by a representative of the Labour Inspectorate in conjunction with the pathologist. The pathologist presents a report with the cause of death to the police. On this evidence together with the circumstances, the Labour Inspectorate will decide whether to pursue the investigation through the criminal law code, or leave it for civil action to be commenced if there is sufficient evidence.

Finally there is the 'continental system' described by Havard in 1960. In this there is no identifiable executive medico-legal officer, as the intention is only to investigate those deaths which already arouse the suspicions of the police. The liberal influences in the eighteenth and nineteenth centuries on the development of civil law and Rousseau's theory of the 'fundamental decency of the citizen' have led most European countries and their colonies to adopt this system. In the Netherlands the Public Prosecutor appoints the Lijkschouwer to investigate unexplained deaths or cases for cremation, and in Denmark there is the Ligysynsmand, who has a similar duty, but very rarely uses it. The main purpose of this type of medico-legal investigation of sudden death is to find out whether grounds for suspicion exist, but a system which does not begin to operate until suspicion of crime is already present defeats its own purpose. This helps to explain some of the difficulties which are encountered in obtaining autopsies following accidents which have occurred outside British waters.

The importance of a properly conducted inquiry into any fatal accident cannot be over-emphasised: the legal consequences and insurance liabilities can be formidable and no effort should be spared to ensure that the most detailed investigation is carried out. The United Kingdom is fortunate in having a judicial procedure which ensures that any unnatural death is rigorously and publicly investigated, but such a system is rarely encountered elsewhere in the world. When an accidental death occurs outside the United Kingdom, therefore, every effort should be made to send an investigatory team, including a forensic pathologist, to the site of the accident, with a brief to make a comprehensive report. If this is impossible, a thorough investigation and autopsy will be assured if the body or bodies are returned to the United Kingdom, where the coroner of the district into which the bodies are imported has the legal authority to insist on a public inquest. However, when local custom does not allow autopsy it may be possible for the pathologist to record external details before they become altered during transport. In addition proper supervision of embalming is an important aspect prior to shipment of a cadaver to the country of origin.

Personnel

It is essential that the person charged with the medico-legal investigation must be a qualified forensic pathologist who is experienced in the investigation of unnatural death, with adequate resources at his disposal. He will require a proper mortuary with access to X-ray facilities and a supporting forensic laboratory. It is usual for the official in charge of the case (e.g. the coroner) to appoint or approve such a person.

Permission

In Britain, when the order for the autopsy has been given by the coroner or procurator fiscal, the body passes into his custody; only following the conclusion of the investigation is it released to the next of kin. If no statutory authority requires autopsy, then a private autopsy may be performed. In this case, written permission from the next of kin should be obtained when possible, but where this is not feasible, reliable oral permission, later confirmed in writing, is acceptable. In all cases formal identification is required. Elsewhere, the written authority of the next of kin is almost always necessary before an autopsy can be conducted. From the practical aspect, however, in the United Kingdom, the authorisation of an autopsy by the coroner or procurator is paramount and can only be reversed on direct intervention by the Home Secretary.

The Non-Fatal Accident

Claims for permanent or partial disability, pain, suffering and loss of earnings may follow a non-fatal accident, which should be investigated with the same thoroughness as a fatal one, although there may be no mandatory legal requirement to do so. These claims are usually handled through an insurance company, and no communication should be made directly to the individuals concerned as any settlement may be prejudiced.

Accident History

On arrival at the scene of the incident it is mandatory that all recorded data, which should include logbooks, notes and tape recordings, must be taken into safe custody. In the inevitable confusion following an accident it is only too easy for these data to become misplaced. Careful appreciation of this information should be made before proceeding with the investigation. This will not only allow the investigators to formulate an impression of the events at an early stage, but also give some lead as to the initial direction of the investigation. Nonetheless, this must not detract from the fact that an objective and unemotional approach is necessary throughout the inquiry.

It is imperative that a proper and detailed history of the events leading up to the accident is obtained. This may be a difficult and tedious procedure, but if it is not properly performed it can prejudice the whole investigation. In any accident situation, witnesses' accounts are often confused. They can be simplified by establishing a strict chronological plan. All witnesses should be interviewed alone at the earliest possible time after the accident and before they have had an opportunity to compare notes. More accurate descriptions are obtained if witnesses are questioned directly than if they are just asked to submit statements.

At every stage, photography must be used to record the scene and equipment. Ideally, views should be taken from each quarter with a measurement scale appearing in each picture. When a detailed report is being compiled, all original notes must be kept for future reference in court.

A description of the position of the body when first found must be recorded, as this may indicate certain types of mechanical failure. Similarly, any procedures which had to be carried out during the recovery of the body must be known; this is especially relevant where victims have been trapped. At a later stage it may be necessary to reconstruct the accident scene to arrive at a satisfactory explanation.

It has to be strongly emphasised that great care has to be taken in these types of investigation to ensure that there is no conflict between the legal authorities and the company or private investigators, and that no attempt is made to usurp their authority. It is, however, very common for the official authorities to seek help from persons who have the technical knowledge necessary for the proper understanding of the complex nature of such accidents.

The basic principle to be followed is that it is better to accumulate too much information and not to reject the recording of any. Statements by witnesses may be conflicting, and it is in this situation that it will be necessary to re-appraise the information recorded and re-question witnesses. In this case the questions should be framed in a non-incriminating way, but in such a manner as to indicate that further and undisclosed information has come forward. It has to be considered that to those inexperienced in being cross-examined, it is very easy to give the answer which they consider the examiner wishes to have, rather than one which is factual; hence the need for cross-reference. The general demeanour of the witness should be noted, as the credibility of an anxious or agitated witness may be doubtful.

A factor to be considered is that of an accurate time scale, and whether Greenwich Mean Time or local time is used. Greenwich time has the advantage of acting as a standard in a situation where messages and information may spread across several time zones, and thus confusion may be avoided. From this point a chronologically orientated factual account may be accumulated.

Diving Accidents

The foregoing comments apply to the investigation of any fatal accident. The following section refers particularly to diving accidents.

Causes

There is no doubt that there has been a high accident rate in the offshore diving industry. However, the figure quoted by Crockford (1974) of a 50% predicted mortality rate over 20 years has substantially improved since that time, possibly as the result of the implementation of diving regulations. A very good measure of this is the evaluation of the risks by the insurance underwriters. In this, Turvey (1983) and J. Sainsbury (1985, personal communication) emphasise the importance of training, status of company and country in which diving operations take place in determining the risks. Given that these are favourable there may be a loading of only 2% on a life insurance premium.

The definitive cause of death given as a statistic has to be considered as the final marker following a certain sequence of events. It is this sequence of events which produced the accident and which forms such a vital part of an accident investigation. This is especially important where the medical findings are minimal, contradictory or negative. There is also the problem of synergism in the accident situation, in which several small and trivial factors, each of little individual importance, combine together to have a cumulative effect, with a resultant accident situation.

Drowning, for example, is a readily acceptable cause of death, but this must be considered only as a marker point at the end of a series of events. The same principle can be applied to other defined causes of death. This is especially relevant in the proper interpretation of medical conditions in which occlusive changes in vital organs, such as vessels of the heart and brain, may be minimal, but in the work environment may be sufficient to cause incapacity and, in the underwater situation, a fatality.

The types of fatal accident fall into a general pattern, as shown by the series of 55 cases reported by Calder (1979) (Table 10.1). The causes of the cases of asphyxia are given in Table 10.2.

Table 10.1. Causes of fatal accidents (Calder 1979)

Cause	%
Asphyxia	51
Pulmonary	29
Hypothermia	5
Nitrogen narcosis	3
Unknown	7
Acute medical conditions	3

Table 10.2. Causes of fatal asphyxia in diving accidents (Calder 1979)

Cause	%
Drowning	24
Trauma from trapping	6
Foreign body in airways	8
Anoxia	11
Squeeze	2

This experience closely equates to that of Hendry (1978), but with more detailed investigation the number of undetermined causes of death is becoming smaller. Hyperthermia as a cause of death, reported more recently, does not appear in this series.

In the diving situation, logbooks and tapes may be available for examination and should be examined before commencing any interviews. No details should be omitted, and facts such as subjective indications of trivial illness and the time of the last meal should be recorded. A check list can be used so that all aspects are covered.

Accident Check List

1. *Medical History*

    Pre-existing disease
    Recent illness
    Last physical examination

2. *Personal History*

    Diving experience and training
    Previous diving accidents
    Near-accidents

3. *Environment*

    Weather
    Sea state
    Visibility
    Wind
    Temperature:
      At surface
      At working depth
    Hazards:
      Cables
      Rig legs
      Underwater obstructions
      Valves
      Pipes
      Propellers
      Tides
      Currents
      Water jets
      Any explosive demolition in the vicinity

4. *Dive Profile*

    History of recent dives
    Depth and duration
    Current dive profile
    Dive of tender or buddy
    Ascent speed
    Stops and untoward incidents
    Pre-dive events
    Food (alcohol)
    Drugs
    Pre-dive behaviour
    Events in recovery, resuscitation, therapy, recompression

5. *Diving Equipment*

    Suit and gloves
    Helmet
    Valves
    Weight belt
    Gas bottles

Gas mixture and flow rates
Purity of gas
Mask
Buoyancy vest
Depth gauge
Cylinder contents
Safety line

6. *Timings*

Establish precise chronological order

Organisation of Accident Investigation

In the offshore situation, most accidents require the expertise of medical, engineering and technical personnel to arrive at a satisfactory explanation. Calder (1985) has emphasised the necessity of cooperation and teamwork in the investigation of complicated accidents. This is diagrammatically represented for a diving accident in Fig. 10.1.

There needs to be a central coordinator who is usually the coroner or procurator. However, this may be deputed to the Diving Inspector. Usually, as well as the official channels of information, there are other professional bodies which can give constructive information and experience to the investigation. The Association of Offshore Diving Contractors (AODC) representative usually communicates in an ad hoc manner with medical experts from the Diving Medical Advisory Committee (DMAC) or the Decompression Sickness Panel (DCP). These are non-statutory bodies of doctors, scientists and engineers with broad experience in diving matters.

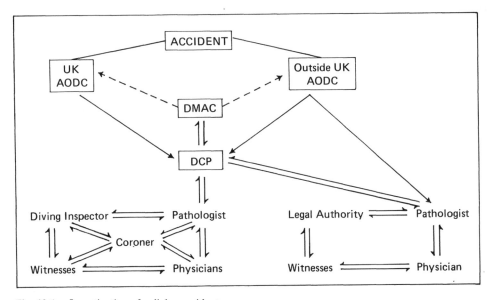

Fig. 10.1. Investigation of a diving accident.

The DMAC is an independent group with a secretariat provided by AODC while the DCP is an element of the Medical Research Council, and can give an objective opinion on the interpretation of data, and methods of approach to the particular accident.

It is to be emphasised that the company concerned in an accident should endeavour to use its own medical personnel to help in the conduct of the investigation. The company also has a right to have a representative at the autopsy.

Recovery, Storage and Preservation of Bodies

Recovery

When death occurs it is obvious that physiological mechanisms cease. Therefore, when death has occurred under pressure, standard decompression schedules are not applicable. However, some attempt must be made to reduce the artefacts which may be produced by a sudden release of pressure causing organs in enclosed cavities to tear. Experience has suggested that once death has been confirmed the body should be left at pressure for 1 h in order to allow the processes of coagulation and lysis to take place, after which it can be reduced at about 100 ft every 15 min, which allows the release of free gas without excessive tissue damage. An excessively slow decompression will allow the processes of decomposition to proceed which, themselves, will distort histological appearances.

Storage

When possible, the cadaver should be sealed in a polythene body bag before storage, as it helps to prevent loss or addition of trace evidence. In addition, the hands should be covered with small polythene bags. This will allow, at a later stage, the examination of scrapings from fingernails which may show retained fragments of the environment indicating precisely the victim's last activity. In addition, it may be possible to identify the presence of products of cannabis on the fingers, should there have been any suspicion of drug taking.

Optimum conditions for preservation are 0°–4°C, and on no account should bodies be frozen below 0°C before autopsy has been performed. Minimal interference should be maintained and the suit left intact. When no refrigeration is available, covering the body with a polythene sheet and surrounding it with ice is sufficient.

Preservation of Specimens

Material for subsequent microscopical examination is preserved in 10% formol saline, and it is to be remembered that approximately 20 times the volume of fixative to tissue is required. A period of 1 week (and in the case of brain, 3 weeks) should elapse to allow fixation before transportation, especially if this is to be by air. The conveyance of human remains by air is governed by the International Air Transport Association Restricted Articles Regulations 1979. Under paragraph 805 it is permitted only to allow 5 l formalin in each container, which itself must be packed in a wooden or fibre box with sufficient surrounding material to absorb the solution in case of spillage. The United States imposes additional conditions on the International Air Transport Association Regulations.

Equipment

After recovery of the body there must be minimal interference with it and its associated equipment. Valves should only be manipulated as far as is necessary to make the apparatus safe. A record must be made of any turns of valves, if necessary marking their position with paint before sealing to await expert technical examination. When gas cylinders are to be sent for laboratory analysis, it should be noted that they cannot be transported by air whilst containing pressurised gas under current Air Transport Freight Regulations.

The body should remain in the suit until the time of autopsy. It is important to relate any marks on the body or suit to the circumstances of the accident (see Figs. 10.2 and 10.3). It is best to cut the suit off the body to avoid any interference with equipment.

Role of the Pathologist

The pathologist's preliminary investigation is to determine how, when, where and by what means death occurred and not to attribute any blame. The pathologist is only able to identify certain definite facts revealed by tissue changes. These, when considered in the light of their history, will allow him to project a reasonable explanation of the fatal events in most cases.

The main aims of the pathologist's examination are to find any medical evidence which might reveal:

1. Natural disease or abnormality which could have caused impaired function and provided a possible or probable medical cause of the accident

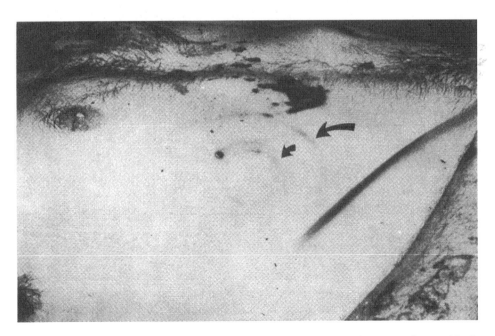

Fig. 10.2. Marks on the chest of a diver who was sucked against the flange of an open valve, resulting in death from traumatic asphyxia.

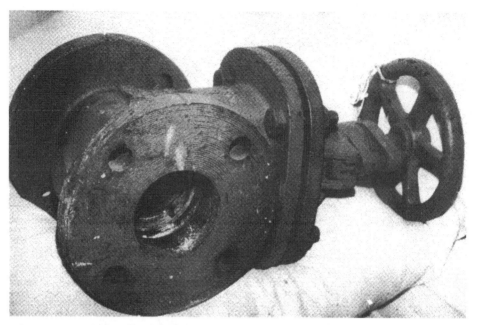

Fig. 10.3. The flange and valve which caused the marks depicted in Fig. 10.2.

2. A possible or probable non-medical cause of the accident
3. The probable events leading up to the accident
4. The probable events at the time immediately after the accident

The fact that a recent medical examination has been performed does not exclude natural disease. Mason (1963) pointed out the presence of severe coronary artery disease which was disclosed at autopsy in apparently fit air crew. It is essential to establish the presence or absence of natural disease, as some minor or trivial medical conditions may contribute to death in the hyperbaric environment. For example, the presence of a trivial respiratory infection may, during a dive, be sufficient to cause blockage of an airway with gas trapping and lung rupture during decompression. As with any other investigation of an unnatural death, the possibility of crime must also not be overlooked. It is important that the medical record of the diver is available to the pathologist in order that findings may be correctly correlated with those found on clinical examination.

Having established the presence or absence of natural disease, the pathologist's next duty is to determine the precise cause of death and relate this to the hyperbaric situation in which it has occurred. This will require him to have a detailed knowledge of the different hyperbaric environments, diving techniques, gas mixtures and decompression procedures.

The direct effects of the hyperbaric environment which may lead to death are gas embolism, pulmonary barotrauma and decompression sickness. Indirectly, death may be caused by toxic gases, drowning or hypo- and hyperthermia. Too often an immediately apparent and acceptable cause of death, such as drowning, may be recorded as the definitive cause when, in fact, this was only the final event and the real causes which led to it are overlooked or disregarded.

Careful examination of the exterior of the body may give the most important clues to the cause of the accident. Figure 10.2 shows the mark on a diver's chest caused by the valve in Figure 10.3. The valve was open and the diver was sucked so hard against it that he was trapped and unable to free himself.

Contributory factors, if not direct causes of death, which leave no mark at autopsy include cold, which produces cardiac arrhythmias, especially in people with myocardial ischaemia (Eldridge 1979; Keating et al. 1980; Schenck and McAnniff 1978). Heating failure in a heliox environment can cause rapid hypothermia.

Oxygen poisoning and nitrogen narcosis also leave no autopsy evidence, though there may be evidence of convulsions from the former. Hyperthermia may also be a cause of death that leaves little trace, though the history should leave little doubt. Drowning may be the end-result of alternobaric vertigo or a 'vestibular bend' which may occur when bubbles form in the inner ear as a result of decompression or gas changes.

The presence of gas bubbles in the tissue does not necessarily indicate that they are related to decompression, far less that they were a contributory cause of death. Nevertheless their presence must be correctly interpreted; the electron microscope technique advocated by Richter et al. (1978) may be helpful.

The fact that the diver was receiving gas is no guarantee that he was not short of oxygen. The presence of Tardieu spots, with purple discoloration of the skin, suggests an anoxic death, while a rosy pink appearance of the skin is indicative of carbon monoxide poisoning.

Autopsy Technique

It is not appropriate to describe the details of a specific technique in this monograph, for each case may demand a specific and individual approach dictated by circumstances. It is, however, imperative that the correct interpretation is placed on the finding of bubbles and free gas within body cavities and tissues. This must be carefully evaluated, either as part of the accident complex, or arising as an artefact.

This can only be achieved by a basic knowledge of hyperbaric physiology, a detailed history of the accident and close cooperation with a physician with specialist knowledge of diving medicine. In practical terms the philosophy adopted in the Memorandum on the Investigation of Civil Air Accidents, published by the Department of Trade and Industry in 1971 has been found to be a useful basis.

Unascertainable Cause of Death

With the exclusion of identifiable causes of death, there is a residuum of cases in which the fact of cardiac arrest is the only certain pathological finding. It is in this type of case that reasoned consideration of the facts by the investigating team can lead to the establishment of a reasonable cause for the accident. However, in some cases it may be preferable to admit that the precise cause of the accident is unknown rather than propose a theoretical explanation on inadequate evidence, only to be proved wrong at a later date when more data become available.

Laboratory Support in Diving Accidents

Gas

Gas samples from the body are of no value after death in determining the purity of the respired gases. However, it is mandatory that samples of breathing mixture are analysed. Much depends on the quality and facilities of the local laboratories as to the reliability of the results and, where possible, samples should be submitted to laboratories experienced in this type of work, such as the Admiralty Marine Technology Establishment (Physiological Laboratory) at Alverstoke. Nonetheless, this may be difficult from foreign parts because, as already mentioned, the transport of pressurised gas bottles by air is prohibited under air cargo regulations.

Body Fluid Samples

The standard sampling procedure is used:

Blood.   Aliquots from leg veins should be transferred to clean dry containers. Standard analyses for drugs and carbon monoxide should be performed. Fluoride containers are used for blood alcohol estimation, which should also be done routinely. If samples are obtained very shortly after death, right and left heart blood may be of value for the determination of drowning by means of electrolyte estimation, as suggested by Modell (1971). For this, preservation is in lithium heparin.

Urine.   A clean sample should be taken for analysis for alcohol and basic and acidic drugs.

Cerebrospinal Fluid and Vitreous Humour.   These fluids when properly preserved and subsequently analysed may be helpful in establishing electrolyte imbalance, and should be taken into fluoride and lithium heparin.

Bile.   A sample of bile must be taken in any case where morphine-like drugs may be suspected.

Stomach Contents.   These should be taken into a sealed container.

Bone Marrow.   A clean sample of bone marrow taken into a clean, dry container may be of help in establishing a case of drowning. The diatoms which are resistant to decomposition in the marrow are compared with those in the water where death occurred, and 1 l of water taken from the site and at the depth at which death occurred is also necessary.

By use of these standard sampling techniques it should be possible to identify most stable drugs and metabolic products. In addition, the products of marijuana, in the form of cannabinoids in the blood and urine, can be identified for up to 1 week after indulgence, and the distillation products on the fingers, after several days of immersion in water (Marks et al. 1976). It must be considered that negative findings in toxicological screening are equally as valuable as positive ones.

Transport of Bodies

Where possible, the services of an undertaker with experience in this field should be sought, but in may parts of the world no such people exist. Therefore a brief outline of the procedures to be adopted may be helpful.

Return of a Body to the United Kingdom

A medical certificate giving the cause or circumstances of death must be obtained from the appropriate authorities, who will also give written authorisation for export of the body. Several copies of such documents should be made immediately. For air transportation the body has to be embalmed before being sealed in a zinc-lined box. Embalming may have to be performed by a medical officer where local custom dictates. On arrival in the United Kingdom the body passes into the custody of the coroner in whose area it is imported. The coroner will decide whether to order an autopsy. The foreign certificate is usually acceptable to the Registrar of Births, Marriages and Deaths of the district in which burial is to take place. A certificate of No Liability to Register is issued, giving authorisation for burial. When cremation is required the procedure can become more complicated. The foreign certificate may not be acceptable to the medical referee of the crematorium, who may then require an autopsy or have the case reported to the coroner for autopsy. In the former case Form D and the latter Form E, is issued under the Cremation Acts 1902 and 1952 as the medical certificate.

Export of Bodies from the United Kingdom

Embalming and sealing in a zinc-lined coffin is still necessary. An 'Out of England Certificate' from the coroner is required for authorisation to be obtained from the Home Office to allow the body to leave the country. A similar procedure holds in Scotland, involving the procurator fiscal and the Scottish Home and Health Department. In addition, some countries require a certificate stating that no infectious or communicable disease was present at the time of death.

Conclusion

Even in the most obvious of accidents it behoves the investigators to accumulate all the data possible. As a result of such an approach it may be possible to utilise scanty data with previous experience to establish the cause of the tragedy and prevent a future recurrence.

Bibliography

Calder IM (1979) Fatal underwater accidents. Univ Microfilm, Michigan, pp 163–166
Calder IM (1985) A method for investigating specialised accidents with special reference to diving. Forensic Sci Int 27: 119–127
Cox RAF, King J, McIver NKI, Calder IM (1980) Hyperthermia. Lancet II: 1309
Crockford GW (1974) A four-year survey of mortality in divers. Eighth Symposium, Polytechnic of North London, 20–21 September, pp 178–182

Eldridge L (1979) Proceedings of International Conference on Underwater Education, Houston, October

Findley TP (1977) An autopsy protocol for skin and scuba diving deaths. Am J Clin Pathol 67: 440–443

Goad RD, (1981) Medical aspects of amateur diving — discussion. VII Annual Congress of the European Undersea Biomedical Society, Cambridge pp 104–112

Goldhahn RT (1976) Scuba diving death: A review and approach for the pathologist. Legal Medicine Annual. Forensic Science Division, Armed Forces Institute of Pathology, Washington.

Havard JDJ (1960) Detection of secret homicide. Macmillan, London (Cambridge studies in criminology, vol II)

Hendry WT (1978) The offshore scene and it hazards. In: Mason JK (ed) Pathology of violent injury. Edward Arnold, Illinois, pp 297–317

Keating WR, Hayward MG, McIver NKI (1980) Hypothermia during saturation diving in the North Sea. Br Med J 280: 291

McAnniff JJ, Schenck HV (1974) Investigation of scuba deaths. J Sports Med 2: 199–208

Marks J, Teale JD, King LJ (1976) Radioimmunoassay of cannabis products in blood and urine. In: Nahas GG (ed) Marijuana: chemistry, biochemistry and cellular effects. Springer New York

Mason JK (1963) Asymptomatic disease of coronary arteries in young men. Br Med J II: 1234

Mobon D (1977) Revised figures for diving fatalities. Dept of Energy, January 13th, Ref 17

Modell JH (1971) Pathophysiology and treatment of drowning and near-drowning. Thomas, Springfield

Occupational Health (1976) Why these divers died. (Editorial) Occup Health 28: 343–347

Richter K, Loblich HJ, Wyllie JW (1978) Ultrastructural aspects of bubble formation in human fatal accidents after exposure to compressed air. Virchows Arch [Pathol Anat] 380: 261–271

Schenck HV, McAnniff JJ (1978) United States underwater fatality statistics 1976. US Department of Commerce National Oceanic Atmospheric Administration, Washington

Turvey PJ (1983) Diving: A background and guide to the assessment of risk. Swiss Reinsurance Company (UK), London

Appendix 1

Recommended Drugs and Dressings for Offshore Installation Sick Bays

Drugs

*These items will be required under the new Offshore Installations and Pipeline Works First-Aid Regulations in United Kingdom Waters when they come into effect.
†These items should not be carried on installations where there is no qualified medic

Medication	Recommended for	Special instructions/ labelling	Quantities for installations or barges where the following numbers are regularly at work		
			1–25	26–100	101 or more

Analgesics

Medication	Recommended for	Special instructions/ labelling	1–25	26–100	101 or more
Soluble aspirin and codeine tabs. BP 500 mg	Pain	Dissolve in water	100	250	1000
Soluble aspirin	Pain and fevers	Dissolve in water	100	250	1000
*Paracetamol tabs.	Relief of minor pain	Store in airtight container	50	500	1000
Dextropropoxyphene and paracetamol tabs.	Relief of more severe pain		50	250	500
†*Dihydrocodeine tartrate tabs.	Relief of more severe pain	30-mg tabs.	25	50	100
†*Inj. morphine sulph. 15 mg in 1 ml	Relief of severe pain; shock	Check expiry date	6	6	20
*Inj. pethidine 100 mg in 2 ml	Relief of severe pain; shock	Check expiry date	6	6	20

Antibiotics

Medication	Recommended for	Special instructions/ labelling	1–25	26–100	101 or more
*Caps. ampicillin 250 mg	Infections	Check expiry date	25	100	250
*Tabs. co-trimoxazole	Infections	Check expiry date	25	100	250
*Caps. penicillin V (or tabs.) 250 mg	Infections	Check expiry date	25	100	250
†*Inj. pencillin soluble (forte)	Infections	Check expiry date, do not use more than 24 h after adding water	6 amps.	10 amps.	20 amps.
Inj. ampicillin 500 mg	Prevention of secondary drowning. To be given intramuscularly	Check expiry date	2 amps.	2 amps.	2 amps.
*Tabs. tetracycline 250 mg	Infections	Check expiry date	25	100	250
*Tabs. erythromycin	Infections	Use in persons sensitive to penicillin	25	100	250

Medication	Recommended for	Special instructions/ labelling	Quantities for installations or barges where the following numbers are regularly at work		
			1–25	26–100	101 or more

Alimentary preparations

*Aluminium hydrox. tabs. 500 mg	Indigestion	Chew before swallowing	100	250	1000
Tabs. diphenoxylate HCl with atropine sulph.	Diarrhoea		100	250	500
Tabs. hyoscine HBr 0.3 mg	Seasickness		20	50	100
† Tabs. metoclopramide monohydro-chloride	Gastritis		20	50	100
Mist. kaolin et morph.	Diarrhoea	Check expiry date	100 ml	250 ml	500 ml
Tabs senna BP	Constipation		25	50	100
Anusol suppos.	Haemorrhoids		10	20	50
† Inj. promethazine HCl 25 mg/ml	Severe vomiting; severe allergies		3 amps.	6 amps.	10 amps.
Mist mag. trisil.	Indigestion	Check expiry date	100 ml	250 ml	500 ml

Antihistamines

*Tabs. prometha-zine HCl 10 mg	Allergies	May cause drowsiness; keep patient under observation and not at work	25	50	100
Tabs. chlorphenir-amine maleate 4 mg	Allergies		25	50	100

Aural preparations

Neomycin, polymyxin, hydrocortisone ear drops	Otitis externa	Check expiry date	2 bottles	6 bottles	10 bottles
Paradichloro-benzene, chlor-butol and turpentine ear drops	Softening wax	Check expiry date	1 bottle	1 bottle	1 bottle

Nasal preparations

Xylometazoline HCl drops 0.1%	Relief of nasal congestion	Check expiry date	3 bottles	6 bottles	12 bottles
*Inhalant caps.	Colds and respiratory congestion		50	100	200

Medication	Recommended for	Special instructions/labelling	Quantities for installations or barges where the following numbers are regularly at work		
			1–25	26–100	101 or more

Local anaesthetics

Medication	Recommended for	Special instructions/labelling	1–25	26–100	101 or more
†*Lignocaine gel 2%	Catheterisation/ intubation	Sterile; 25-ml tubes	1	2	6
†*Lignocaine HCL 1%	Wound suturing	2-ml amps. must not contain adrenaline	10	20	50

Miscellaneous preparations

Medication	Recommended for	Special instructions/labelling	1–25	26–100	101 or more
*Lip salve	Dry cracked lips		12	50	100
*Magnesium sulph. paste	Treatment of minor infected lesions	4-oz containers	2	4	6
*Plaster solvent	Removal of plaster adhesive	Keep tightly closed	0.5 l	1 l	2 l
*White soft paraffin	Protective preparation		0.5 kg	1 kg	1 kg
†*Plasma expanders	Intravenous fluid	Store in dark, dry conditions below 25°C; 500-ml containers; check expiry date	10	20	50
*Water for injection BP		Check expiry date	20	100	100
Surgical spirit		External use only	150 ml	250 ml	500 ml
Methyl salicylate liniment BPC	Muscle strains	External use only	100 ml	250 ml	500 ml
†Inj. tetanus toxoid	Prophylactic in contaminated wounds		3	6	10
†Tabs. glyceryl trinitrate	Angina pectoris		20	50	100

Ophthalmic preparations

Medication	Recommended for	Special instructions/labelling	1–25	26–100	101 or more
*Fluorescein drops 2% (minims)	Staining eyes	Individual single-dose amps.	20 amps.	50 amps.	100 amps.
*Saline 0.9% drops	Removal of excess fluorescein	Individual single-dose amps.	20 amps.	50 amps.	100 amps.
*Chloramphenicol ophthalmic ointment	Eye infections	Single-dose containers; check expiry date	25	100	250
*Oxybuprocaine BP 0.4%	Relief of pain after eye injury	Single-dose containers; check expiry date	25	50	200
Homatropine eye drops	Dilation of pupil	Single-dose containers; check expiry date	10	20	30

Medication	Recommended for	Special instructions/ labelling	Quantities for installations or barges where the following numbers are regularly at work		
			1–25	26–100	101 or more
Welder's eye drops (adren. acid. tart. 0.095% zinc sulph. BP 0.25%; buric acid BP 3.4%; phenol mercuric acid as preservative 0.002%)	'Arc eye'	Keep in well-sealed containers	10 ml	3 × 10 ml	6 × 10 ml
Sulphacetamide eye drops BPC 10%	Eye infections	Keep in well-sealed containers	3 × 10 ml	6 × 10 ml	12 × 10 ml

Oral and dental preparations

*Mouthwash solution tabs. BPC	Mouthwash/ gargle	Dissolve 1 tab. in 150 ml warm water	100	250	1000
Benzocaine lozenges	Sore throat		50	100	200
Oil of cloves BP	Toothache	Apply on cotton bud to tooth	1 bottle	1 bottle	1 bottle

Respiratory preparations

†*Terbutaline injection 0.5 mg/ml	Bronchospasm	Check previous exposure	6 amps.	10 amps.	20 amps.
Mist. ipecal. et morph. BPC	Coughs	Check expiry date	250 ml	500 ml	1 l
Opiate squill linctus	Cough suppressant	Check expiry date	100 ml	200 ml	300 ml

Resuscitatory preparations

†*Hydrocortisone sodium phosph. inj. 100 mg in 1 ml	Severe shock	Check expiry date	6 amps.	10 amps.	30 amps.
†*Frusemide 10 mg in 2 ml	Oedema	Check expiry date	3 amps.	6 amps.	6 amps.
†Inj. adrenaline 1/1000 1 ml amps	Anaphylactic shock	Do not give intravenously; check expiry date	3 amps.	6 amps.	10 amps.
Inj. methyl prednisolone 2 g	Prevention of secondary drowning. To be given intravenously	Check expiry date	2 amps.	2 amps.	2 amps.

Sedatives and psychotropics

†*Inj. chlorpromazine 25 mg/ml	Sedation	Check expiry date	3 amps.	5 amps.	10 amps.

Medication	Recommended for	Special instructions/ labelling	Quantities for installations or barges where the following numbers are regularly at work		
			1–25	26–100	101 or more
†*Inj. diazepam BNF 10 mg	Rapid sedation	Check expiry date	3 amps.	6 amps.	10 amps.
*Tabs. diazepam 5 mg	Sedation		20	50	100
*Caps. temazepam 10 mg	Insomnia		20	50	100

Skin preparations

*Calamine lotion BP	Irritating rashes	External use only	0.5 l	1 l	5 l
*Cetrimide cream 0.5%	Wounds	50-g tubes	3 tubes	6 tubes	20 tubes
*Chlorhexidine gluconate concentrate with cetrimide	Cleaning wounds	25-ml sachets	10 sachets	30 sachets	100 sachets
†Benzoic acid ointment	Some fungal infections	25-g jars	2 × 25 g	6 × 25 g	10 × 25 g
†Benzoyl benzoate application	Scabies	To be applied to whole body except face	200 ml	500 ml	1 l
†Hydrocortisone cream BPC	Allergic rashes	Apply sparingly; 10-g tubes	5 × 10 g	10 × 10 g	20 × 10 g
†Gamma benzene hexachloride 2% in detergent base	Scabies	Shampoo	2 × 50 g	6 × 50 g	10 × 50 g
Zinc ointment BP	Minor wounds	2-oz jars	2 × 2 oz	6 × 2 oz	10 × 2 oz
Zinc, starch and talc dusting powder		10 g	2 × 10 g	6 × 10 g	10 × 10 g
Zinc undecanoate dusting powder	Athlete's foot	10 g	2 × 10 g	6 × 10 g	10 × 10 g
Silver sulphadiazine 1% cream (Flamazine)	Burns	100 g	100 g	4 × 100 g	10 × 100 g

Vitamins

Tabs. ascorbic acid 200 mg	'Colds'		100	250	500
Tabs. Aneur. co (Forte)	'Tonic'		100	250	500

Intravenous fluids

†Haemaccel 500 ml		Steriflex containers	2	6	12
*Macrodex 500 ml		Steriflex containers	2	2	2
†Normal saline 500 ml		Steriflex containers	2	6	12
†Hartmann's solution 500 ml		Steriflex containers	2	4	6

Instruments, Appliances and Sundries

Article	Special requirements	1–25	26–100	101 or more
*Disposable skin cleaners	Sterile, impregnated with isopropyl alcohol; individually wrapped; skin cleansing agent	100 packs	200 packs	300 packs
*Finger stalls	Protective plastic with tapes; large size; 12 to a pack	1 pack	1 pack	1 pack
*†Ryle's tubes	Size 14	1	4	4
*Endotracheal tubes	Cupped McGill type; sizes 7, 7½, 8, 8½, 9; each size	3	3	3
*Resuscitation device	Fitted with non-return valve and angle piece (AMBU bag type)	1	1	1
*Face masks	Standard inflatable pattern; sizes 3, 4, 5, 6; each size	3	3	3
*Airways	Disposable; sizes 2, 3, 4; each size	2	2	2
*Mouth gag	Stainless steel; Ferguson type	1	1	1
*Artery forceps	Spencer Wells; stainless steel	4 pairs	4 pairs	4 pairs
*Forceps	Toothed, dissecting; stainless steel	2 pairs	2 pairs	2 pairs
Forceps	Untoothed, standard and fine	1 pair each	1 pair each	1 pair each
*Scalpel handle	Size 23	1	1	1
*Scalpel blades	Disposable, sterile; individually wrapped; size 23	20	20	20
*Ring saw	Stainless steel	1	1	1
*†Needle holders	Kilner type; stainless steel	1 pack	1 pack	1 pack
*†Sutures	3/0 silk with atraumatic cutting needle; sterile in individual wrappers	12	12	20
	4/0 silk with atraumatic cutting needle; sterile in individual wrappers	12	12	20
*Bowls	Stainless steel 6 in.	1	3	6
*Bowls	Plastic 12–14 in.	1	1	1
*†Suture cutters	Disposable; sterile in individual wrappers	6	6	6
Forceps	Aural; Tilley's	1 pair	1 pair	1 pair
*Scissors	Sharp/blunt; stainless steel; 5 in.	1 pair	1 pair	1 pair
	Blunt/blunt; stainless steel; 5 in.	1 pair	1 pair	1 pair
*Splinter forceps	Hunter's	1 pair	1 pair	1 pair
*Receivers	Stainless steel; 15 cm	1	4	6
	Stainless steel; 25 cm	1	1	1
Vomit bowl	Stainless steel with lid	1	1	1
Gallipots	Stainless steel			
	2 oz	1	1	1
	3 oz	1	1	1
	4 oz	1	1	1
Kidney dish	Stainless steel; 25 cm	1	1	1
Instrument tray	Stainless steel; 22 × 15 × 5 cm	1	1	1
*Measuring jug	Graduated; 0.5 l capacity; polypropylene or stainless steel	1	3	3
*Medicine measure	Graduated; plastic or glass	2	6	6
*Cheatle's forceps and container	Both stainless steel	1	1	1
*Steriliser	Electric; 1 l capacity	1	1	1

Article	Special requirements	Quantities for installations or barges where the following numbers are regularly at work		
		1–25	26–100	101 or more
*†Surgical gloves	Sterile in individual packets; size 7, 7½, 8; disposable	6 pairs	6 pairs	6 pairs
Surgical masks	Disposable	50	50	50
Eye bath	Plastic	3	6	12
Eye undine	Glass	1	1	1
*†Syringes	Disposable; sterile in individual wrappers;			
	2 ml	100	100	100
	5 ml	50	50	50
	10 ml	10	10	10
*†Injection needles	To fit syringes: sterile and individually wrapped;			
	269 × 17 mm	20	100	100
	219 × 14 mm	20	100	100
*†Intravenous infusion sets	Sterile, individually wrapped; Luer fitting	3	3	23
*†Intravenous cannulae	Size 18G (green)	5	10	30
	Size 16G (grey)	5	10	30
*Cervical collar	Sponge rubber; 6.5 × 37 cm or proprietary alternative	2	2	2
*†Eye rod	Glass	2	4	4
*†Stethoscope	Standard type	1	1	1
*†Sphygmomanometer	Aneroid type	1	1	1
*†Laryngoscope	With spare batteries and bulbs; Penlow type with McIntosh blade	1	1	1
*†Diagnostic set	Keeler practitioner type or equivalent with spare batteries and bulbs	1	1	1
*Pen torch	Spare batteries and bulbs	1	2	2
†Patella hammer		1	1	1
*×10 lens magnifier (Berger's loupe)		1	1	1
Tape measure		1	1	1
*Thermometers	Room	1	1	1
	Clinical	2	4	6
	Low reading	2	2	2
*Wooden applicators	100 per box	1 box	1 box	1 box
*Tongue depressors	100 per box	1 box	1 box	1 box
*Reverse-reading Snellen chart		1	1	1
*Suction apparatus	Portable aspirator with mounting tube (foot-operated)	1	1	1
*Suction catheters	Sterile; individually wrapped; size 14, 12; each size	4	4	4
*†Catheters	Foley self-retaining type; in individual wrappers; size 12, 14, 16; each size	2	2	2
	Jacques type; sterile in individual wrapper; size 12, 14, 16; each size	2	2	2
*Spigots or clips	Disposable	12	12	12
*Urine drainage bags	Disposable; sterile	2	2	6
*Urine specimen flasks	Graduated conical; glass/plastic	1	2	2
*Clinistix	Diagnostic agent; bottles of 50 strips; check expiry date	1	2	2

Article	Special requirements	Quantities for installations or barges where the following numbers are regularly at work		
		1–25	26–100	101 or more
*Albustix	Diagnostic agent; bottles of 50 strips; check expiry date	1	2	2
*†Entonox	Cylinder with key attached and corrugated tubing, demand valve, expiratory valve and mouthpiece with disposable plastic masks	6	6	6
*†Oxygen	24-cu ft cylinder of O_2 with key, pressure gauge, flowmeter, angle piece, tubing, mount and suitable disposable face masks	6	6	6
Automatic resuscitator	Volume-cycled machine with manual triggering facility, minimum flow of 100 l/min and capable of delivering 100% O_2	1	1	1
Backboard and special apparatus for spinal injuries		1	1	1
Ship Captain's Medical Guide, Department of Trade, London	Current edition	1	1	1
Offshore Medicine, Springer, Berlin Heidelberg New York	Current edition	1	1	1
*Anti-hypothermia bags	Polyethylene and polyester laminated construction	2	4	4
*†Urethral jelly	Sterile; 8-oz tube	1	2	2
*Hot water bottles	With covers	1	2	2
*Bed pans	Disposable	6	12	12
*Urinals	Disposable	6	12	12
*Stretchers		1	2	2
Stretchers	Collapsible; rescue type with harness and horizontal lifting	1	2	2
*Splints	Wooden	1 set	4 sets	6 sets
Splints	Inflatable	1 set	2 sets	4 sets
Laerdal pocket masks		1	2	4
Safety pins	Assorted	24	48	96
Litmus paper	Red, blue	2 books	2 books	2 books
Tourniquet, Seton	Large	2	4	6
Dental mirror		1	1	1
Acrylic denture repair kit		1	1	1

Dressings

Article	Special requirements	Quantities for installations or barges where the following numbers are regularly at work		
		1–25	26–100	101 or more

Bandages

Article	Special requirements	1–25	26–100	101 or more
Crepe				
5.0 cm		6	12	20
* 7.5 cm		6	12	20
10.0 cm		6	12	20
Elastic adhesive				
5.0 cm		2	6	10
* 7.5 cm		2	6	10
10.0 cm		2	6	10
*Triangular	Individually wrapped; sterile	12	20	20
Open weave		12	12	20
2.5 cm		12	12	20
5.0 cm		12	12	20
7.5 cm		12	12	20
Tubegauze	With applicators			
* size 01		3	10	15
size 12		2	6	10
size 56		2	6	10
* size 34		1	8	12
Tubigrip				
size C		1	2	3
size D		1	2	3

Other Dressings

Article	Special requirements	1–25	26–100	101 or more
*Non-adhesive dressings	Individually wrapped; sterile; perforated film absorbent dressings	1 box	1 box	1 box
*Gauze pads	7.5 × 7.5 cm; sterile; in 5 × 8-ply packs of 5	20 packs	100 packs	300 packs
*Paraffin gauze	Individual paraffin gauze dressings; 100 × 10 cm	2 boxes	6 boxes	10 boxes
*Skin closures	Adhesive; 5 cm length; sterile; individually sealed in envelopes	50	100	100
*Blue waterproof	Assorted sizes with absorbent pad	1 box	1 box	1 box
adhesive plasters	Assorted sizes; non-medicated	1 box	1 box	1 box
Cotton wool rolls				
15 g		6	8	12
25 g		3	4	8
100 g		2	4	6
Cotton wool balls	In sterile packs of 5	20 packs	50 packs	100 packs
Wound dressings	Sterile; air-permeable adhesive waterproof dressing strips with non-medicated absorbent pad; individually wrapped; size			
	7.5 × 1.25 cm;	1 box	4 boxes	5 boxes
	box of 100 assorted sizes	1 box	2 boxes	3 boxes
Waterproof adhesive dressing strip	Individually wrapped; sterile; 6 × 100 cm	3	6	12

Article	Special requirements	Quantities for installations or barges where the following numbers are regularly at work		
		1–25	26–100	101 or more
Standard dressings	Individually wrapped; sterile			
No. 13		6	12	20
No. 14		6	12	20
No. 15		6	12	20
*Hypoallergenic tape	Waterproof, adhesive tape; should			
1.25 cm	not be affected by excessive cold	1	4	6
2.5 cm		1	4	6
Absorbent gauze	non-sterile; 100 m	1	1	1
Absorbent ribbon	1 cm			
gauze		1	1	1
*Dressing towels	Individually wrapped; 2-ply; sterile; absorbent paper towel 50 × 45 cm	10	50	50
*Eye pads	Sterile; individually wrapped	20	20	20
Zinc oxide plaster BPC				
1.0 cm		4	6	10
2.5 cm		4	6	10
5.0 cm		4	6	10
Standard dressings	Individually wrapped; extra large	12	20	40
Roehampton burn				
dressings		12	20	40
Shell dressings		4	8	10
Scrotal supports				
Medium		2	2	2
Large		2	2	2

Appendix 2

Scale III. The Merchant Shipping (Medical Stores) Regulations 1986, SI 1986 No. 144

Part 1: Medicines

Name of medicine	Ordering size	Quantities required
Activated charcoal Activated charcoal effervescent granules	5 g sachet	2
Adrenaline Adrenaline acid tartrate injection 1.8 mg in 1 ml (1 in 1000)	0.5 ml ampoule	5
Aluminium acetate Aluminium acetate ear drops 13%	10 ml bottle with dropper	2
Anaesthetic eye drops Amethocaine 0.5%	In single dose applicator	20
Arachis oil Arachis (peanut) oil	10 ml bottle with dropper	1
Aspirin Dispersible aspirin	300 mg dispersible tablet	200
Atropine Atropine sulphate injection 1 mg in 1 ml	1 ml ampoule	5
Benzoic acid Benzoic acid compound ointment (benzoic acid 6%; salicylic acid 3%; in emulsifying ointment) often called Whitfield's ointment	50 g	1
Benzylpenicillin Benzylpenicillin sodium injection powder (for reconstitution) in a rubber-capped and metal-topped glass vial	600 mg vial	5
Bismuth subgallate Bismuth subgallate compound suppository (bismuth subgallate 200 mg; zinc oxide 120 mg)	1 g suppository	12
Burn cream Silver sulphadiazine cream 1% w/w	50 g tube	4
Calamine lotion Calamine 15% lotion	100 ml bottle	2
Cetrimide concentrate Cetrimide concentrate 40%	100 ml bottle	2

Name of medicine	Ordering size	Quantities Required
Chloramphenicol Chloramphenicol eye ointment 1%	4 g dispenser	2
Chlorpheniramine Chlorpheniramine maleate	4 mg tablet	25
Chlorpromazine Chlorpromazine hydrochloride	25 mg tablet	50
Codeine linctus Codeine phosphate 15 mg in 5 ml linctus	200 ml bottle	2
Compound thymol glycerin Thymol glycerin compound mouthwash (thymol 0.05%; glycerol 10% in water)	200 ml bottle	1
Co-trimoxazole Co-trimoxazole (sulphamethoxazole 400 mg; trimethoprim 80 mg)	480 mg tablet	50
Diazepam Diazepam	5 mg tablet	10
Dihydrocodeine Dihydrocodeine tartrate	30 mg tablet	50
Erythromycin Erythromycin	250 mg tablet	50
Gamma benzene hexachloride Gamma benzene hexachloride 1% body cream	50 g container	2
Gamma benzene hexachloride 2% hair application	50 ml container	1
Glyceryl trinitrate Glyceryl trinitrate	0.5 mg tablet	100
Hydrocortisone ointment Hydrocortisone 1% ointment	15 g container	2
Hydrogen peroxide Hydrogen peroxide 6% solution	100 ml bottle	1
Hyoscine hydrobromide Hyoscine hydrobromide	0.3 mg tablet	50
Lignocaine Lignocaine hydrochloride 1% (plain) 20 mg in 2 ml	2 ml ampoule	5
Magnesium trisilicate Magnesium trisilicate (magnesium trisilicate 250 mg; dried aluminium hydroxide gel 120 mg)	370 g compound tablet	100
Menthol and benzoin Menthol and benzoin inhalation (menthol 1 g; benzoin inhalation to 50 ml)	50 ml bottle	1
Metronidazole Metronidazole	200 mg tablet	20
Morphine Morphine sulphate injection 15 mg in 1 ml	1 ml ampoule	5
Nitrazepam Nitrazepam	5 mg tablet	30
Oil of cloves Clove oil	10 ml bottle	1

Name of medicine	Ordering size	Quantities Required
Paracetamol Paracetamol	500 mg tablet	200
Penicillin V Phenoxymethylpenicillin	250 mg tablet	100
Petroleum jelly Soft paraffin	50 g container	1
Potassium permanganate Potassium permanganate crystals	10 g container	1
Salbutamol Salbutamol aerosol inhaler unit, giving 100 μg per metered inhalation	200 dose container	1
Sodium chloride and dextrose Sodium chloride and dextrose oral powder, compound (35 mmol Na^+; 20 mmol K^+; 37 mmol Cl^-; 18 mmol HCO_3^-; 200 mmol dextrose per litre when reconstituted)	22 g sachets	20
Water for injection Water for injection	2 ml ampoule	5
Zinc ointment Zinc oxide 15% in a simple ointment	25 g container	1

Part 2: Instruments, Appliances and Measuring Equipment

Name of item and ordering description	Quantities required
Canvas roll for instruments To contain the surgical instruments	1
Eye loop Disposable, of nylon with wooden handle	2
Fluorescein strips Fluorescein sodium 1% paper eye test strips	15
Forceps Stainless steel throughout	
Dissecting 12.5 cm	1
Epilation with oblique ends 12.5 cm	1
Spencer Wells 12.5 cm	2
Guerdel airway Conforming to British Standards Institution Standard BS 2927 published on 29.11.57	
Size 4	2
Kidney dish Size 250 mm, conforming to British Standards Institution Standard BS 1823 published on 15.6.73 for stainless steel, or British Standards Institution Standard BS 5452 published on 28.2.77 for sterilisable plastic	1
Lotion bowl Size at least 200 × 90 mm, to BS 1823 for stainless steel, or to BS 5452 for sterilisable plastic, to be lettered 'medical' (for BS standards see entry above for kidney dish)	1

Name of item and ordering description	Quantities required
Magnifying glass 7.5 cm diameter, on handle	1
Measures Dispensing measure, size 10 ml, glass, in 1 ml divisions starting at 1 ml, conforming to British Standards Institution Standard BS 1922 published on 23.1.69	1
Measuring spoon, size 5 ml, plastic, conforming to British Standards Institution Standard BS 3221/6 1985	30
Neck collar Adjustable, fractured (etc.) neck — adult size. Set of 3: small, medium and large	1
Razor Disposable, pack of 5	1
Resuscitator, mouth to mouth Short oral airway with non-return valve, of the Brook airway type	2
Scalpel and blade set Blades and scalpels size 23, sterile, disposable	1
Scissors Stainless steel throughout. Size about 18 cm, one blade sharp-pointed and the other round-ended; conforming to British Standards Institution Standard BS 3646 published on 19.7.63	1
Splints Set of common splints	1
Inflatable splint, set of 4 (half-leg, full-leg, half-arm, full arm)	1
Liston's thigh splint 140 cm	1
Suture and needle pack Sterile, non-absorbable, sutures BP, of monofilament nylon, or silk, swaged to a 26 mm and 40 mm half-circle needle, with a cutting edge. Each needle and suture to be in a sealed pack	
26 mm half-circle needle	3
40 mm half-circle needle	3
Sterile, absorbable sutures BP, of catgut swaged to a 40 mm half-circle cutting needle	1
Syringe and needle, hypodermic pack Sterile, disposable, conforming to British Standards Institution Standard BS 5801 published on 30.6.76. Each syringe and needle in a sealed pack	
2 ml syringe with a 0.8 mm (21 SWG) × 4 cm needle	20
Thermometers — including hygrometers To give the temperature in °C, or °C and °F. Each thermometer, with instructions as to its use, to be in a strong metal or strong plastic case, and to conform to British Standards Institution Standard BS 691 published on 31.12.79	
Ordinary range clinical thermometer, stubby bulb pattern	2
Sub-normal range, low body temperature thermometer, stubby bulb pattern	1
Urine testing equipment Salicylsulphonic acid 20% w/v, in a 25 ml bottle	2

Part 3: Bandages, Cotton Wool and Dressings

Name of item and ordering description	Quantities required
Bandages	
Each bandage to be individually wrapped	
Crepe, BP, 7.5 cm × 4.5 m when stretched	3
Elastic adhesive, BP, 7.5 cm × 4 m	2
Triangular, calico, BP, with 2 sides of about 90 cm and a base of about 127 cm	4
Tubular gauze bandage, seamless, of a size suitable for finger dressings, a length of 20 m with applicator	1
Conforming bandage, 5 cm × 3.5 m BP	4
Conforming bandage, 7.5 cm × 3.5 m BP	6
Butterfly closures	
Adhesive skin closures, length approximately 5 cm, individually sealed sterile in a container	10
Cotton wool	
Absorbent cotton and viscose wadding, BP, in a roll, in damp-proof packaging	
Package containing 15 g, sterile	8
Package containing 100 g, unsterile	2
Dressings	
All dressings are to be individually wrapped and in a strong and suitable container	
Sterile paraffin gauze dressings, BP, size 10 × 10 cm individually wrapped	20
Standard BPC dressings	
The containers for these dressings should each bear a label with instructions covering the following points: 'Open by pulling tab. Avoid touching wound and do not finger the face of the sterilised pad. Place pad over wound, retain hold of short end of bandage, wind remainder firmly and tie in a knot'	
Small plain wound dressing standard no. 13 BPC	4
Medium plain wound dressing, standard no. 14 BPC	4
Large plain wound dressing, standard no. 15 BPC	4
Dressing strip	
Elastic adhesive medicated dressing strip BPC, 6 cm × 1 m in a packet	1
Gauze	
Packet containing one piece of sterile absorbent cotton gauze BP, size 30 × 90 cm	7
Gauze pads	
Packet containing 5 sterile gauze pads BP size 7.5 × 7.5 cm	7
Gauze ribbon	
Packet containing sterile absorbent cotton gauze ribbon BP, size 2.5 cm × 5 m	1
Suspensory bandage	
Large size	1
Zinc oxide tape	
Zinc oxide plaster BP, 2.5 cm × 5 m, on a spool	1

Part 4: Sundries and Publications

Name of item and ordering description	Quantities required
Bag, body Large size, designed to hold a dead person in a refrigerator up to 14 days or in a cool place up to 5 days	1
Buds Of viscose or cotton wool, in a container	20
Disinfectant To conform to the specification for disinfectant prescribed in Schedule 4, Part 1	3
Eye baths	1
Eye pads Sterile	2
Finger stalls With tapes, of robust material throughout, two or more sizes	5

First aid kit
To be distributed around the ship
The following to be in a damp-proof strong canvas bag, satchel, or box, with a strap for carrying:
  8 calico, triangular, bandages BP, with sides of about 90 cm and a base of about 127 cm
  2 standard dressings no. 13 BPC
  2 standard dressings no. 14 BPC
  2 standard dressings no. 15 BPC
  12 medium size safety pins
  30 assorted elastic adhesive dressing strips medicated BPC
	2

Insecticide To conform to the specifications for insecticides prescribed in Schedule 4 Part 2 In powder form — in an air-tight container	100 g
Labels Tags for patients who have been given morphine	5
Nail brush Of strong sterilisable plastic throughout	1
Safety pins Rustless, size 5 cm	12
Stretcher Neil-Robertson type	1

Publications
  Ship Captain's Medical Guide — current edition
  DOT form SCMG/3, visit to doctor form
  A copy of the regulations referred to in this notice
  A copy of this notice and subsequent amendments
  Controlled drugs register
	1
	10
	1
	1
	1

Appendix 3

Drugs and Medical Equipment to be Kept at Diving Sites

1. The following lists are comprehensive and include all items which could be required by a doctor attending a diving-related illness, assuming that he has no equipment with him on arrival at the site. They include equipment which may be needed for the treatment of decompression illness or its complications, and which should be kept separately, under the responsibility of the Diving Supervisor. They do *not* include all drugs, dressings or equipment which may be needed for all other non-diving related conditions, such as intercurrent illnesses or trauma. The medical materials for those situations are legally required to be held in the vessel or installation's hospital (see Appendix 1).

   The drugs, dressings and equipment specified are for use by a specialist doctor who may be called to the scene, or for use by an emergency medical technician under the direction of a medical specialist, either on site or over the radio, in the treatment of decompression illness or its complications. (However, see also 3 below.)

2. This equipment should be available at all offshore diving sites. It will be appreciated, however, that individual contractors may wish to modify the lists, depending on the circumstances and location of the work in hand, on the medical support which has been agreed or on the advice of their doctor or medical adviser.

   If some of the medical equipment is available (e.g. in the sickbay of a diving support vessel) or if more than one diving operation is being conducted at a site, then it is not necessary to duplicate the equipment for each separate activity or operation. However, arrangements should exist to ensure that there is ready access to the equipment for both or all operations in the event of it being needed.

3. The equipment should be stowed in a double-locked container and labelled 'Normally to be opened only on the instructions of a doctor', except for those items marked with an asterisk, '*', which could be stored in a separate container to be available for general first aid purposes.

   In practice it is more convenient if the equipment in the overall list is broken into specific packages as follows:

   Pack 1. Medical equipment to be held within a diving bell
   Pack 2. Medical equipment to be held within a deck compression chamber
   Pack 3. Respiratory and resuscitation equipment
   Pack 4. Intravenous cut-down, suturing and arrest of haemorrhage equipment
   Pack 5. Intravenous infusion equipment (all drugs, including resuscitation drugs, should be labelled 'Normally to be opened only on the advice of a doctor')
   Pack 6. Diagnostic equipment
   Pack 7. Sterile thoracocentesis — 'chest drain' equipment (should be labelled 'Normally to be opened only on the advice of a doctor')

Pack 8. Urinary catheterisation equipment (should be labelled 'Normally to be opened only on the advice of a doctor')

Pack 9. Sundry first aid equipment and dressings.

4. Concern has been expressed over the security of controlled drugs ('DDAs'), and morphine may be omitted if security cannot be guaranteed. Checks should, however, be made to ensure that such drugs are available nearby for use in an emergency, e.g. in the installation's sick bay.

5. In some countries, regulations require that specific medical equipment, which is itemised in the regulations, should be held at the site of a diving operation. Clearly in such cases, regulations take precedence over this or any other guidance note.

Complete List of Medical Equipment to be held at the Site of an Offshore Diving Operation

Surgical Equipment and Instruments

2	Small dressing bowls
1	Self-retaining Foley type catheter SR size 16 (pre-sterilised)
1	Self-retaining Foley type catheter SR size 18 (pre-sterilised)
4	Catheter spigots
2	20 ml amps. sterile water
2	Sterile urinary drainage bags
3	Intravenous giving sets with long drip chambers (e.g. Baxter)
5	20 ml syringes
2	5 ml syringes
2	2 ml syringes
5	No. 21 1½ in. (3.5 cm) hypodermic needles
5	No. 25 1 in. (2.5 cm) hypodermic needles
1	Laerdal resuscitator bag with a 100% oxygen fitting and with fitting to BIBS
1	Laerdal pocket mask
4	Medicut cannulae size 16
4	Medicut cannulae size 18
2	Butterfly infusion sets 19G
4	Plastic bottle holders
1	Laryngoscope and batteries
1	No. 9 endotracheal tube
1	No. 9.5 endotracheal tube
1	Oesophageal obturator airway
2	Disposable oropharyngeal airway size 3
2	Disposable oropharyngeal airway size 4
4 *	Tourniquet (large)
4	Mouth-to mouth resuscitator (Brook airway professional model)
3	Pair 7 in. (12.5 cm) Mayo scissors
2	Foot-operated suckers
3	Fine endotracheal suckers
2	Yankauer suckers (wide bore)

2   Mouth gags
9   Pairs Spencer Wells artery forceps: 6 pairs 12 cm (5 in.); 3 pairs 18 cm (7 in.)
2   Sequestrene bottles
4   Plain blood bottles
1   Drip stand or hook
1   Sterilised 'cut-down' kit containing:
           Disposable scalpel
           2 scalpel blades
           1 pair pointed scissors
           1 pair toothed dissecting forceps
           1 pair fine-toothed dissecting forceps
           2 pairs mosquito forceps
           1 aneurysm needle
           1 small retractor
           1 pair needle holders
           2 × 2/0 catgut plain on atraumatic needles   )   (in packs
           2 × 0   catgut plain on atraumatic needles   }   attached to
           4 × 3/0 black silk on atraumatic needles   )   exterior)

Dressings

5   Pairs sterile disposable gloves, large
20   Sealed alcohol swabs for cleaning skin
3   * Rolls 1 in. (2.5 cm) adhesive tape (Elastoplast)
2   Tubes sterile urethral anaesthetic gel and nozzle
1   Short arm splint (board for i.v.)
2   * 3 in. (7.5 cm) crepe bandages
2   * 1 in. (2.5 cm) rayon porous synthetic adhesive tape
100* Sterile gauze swabs (20 packets of 5); 5 packets to be placed with chest drain
       set)
1   * 1 in. (2.5 cm) roll gauze tape
100* Sterile cotton wool balls (20 packets of 5); 5 packets to be placed with chest
       drain set)
2   * Sterile standard dressing packs, large
2   * Sterile standard dressing packs, medium
2   * Sterile standard dressing packs, small
4   Dressings (Shell or Field), large
6   * Triangular bandages
1   Tube lubricating jelly
12   * Safety pins, various sizes
15   * Adhesive dressings, various sizes
1   * Tube cetrimide 0.5% cream

Drugs

4   10 ml 1% Xylocaine (1 to be placed with chest drain set)
10   * 10 ml Savlon sachets (or chlorhexidine 1% solution; 2 sachets to be placed with
       chest drain set)

2   500 ml bottle dextran 70 in saline
2   1 l bottles dextrose saline
4   500 ml bottles normal saline
1   250 ml mannitol 10%
1   5 ml heparin injection 5000 units/ml
4   Diazepam injections 10 mg in 2 ml
5   Diazepam tablets 5 mg
5   2 ml dexamethasone injections 4 mg/ml
20   Dexamethasone tablets 2 mg
10   Injections soluble hydrocortisone 100 mg (i.v. or i.m.)
2   2 ml frusemide injections 10 mg/ml
2   2 ml prochlorperazine injections 12.5 mg/ml
2   1 ml chlorpheniramine injections 10 mg/ml
2   10 ml adrenaline injections 1:10 000
2   10 ml calcium gluconate injections 10%
2   Atropine injections 0.6 mg/ml
4   50 ml sodium bicarbonate 8.4% solution (1 m equiv./ml)
25   Cinnarizine tablets
1   Bottle soluble dextrose tablets
25 * Soluble aspirin tablets
1   50 g silver sulphadiazine cream 1%
3   Morphine sulphate injections 15 mg in 2 ml (subject to double-locked storage)

Diagnostic Instruments

1   Pencil torch with batteries
1   Thermocouple thermometer or means of measuring temperature
1   Stethoscope
1   Aneroid sphygmomanometer with a hole drilled in the outer case
1   Auriscope with spare batteries and ophthalmic eyepiece
1   Tuning fork 128 Hz
1   Tuning fork 512 Hz
1   Bottle urine testing strips (Haemocombistix)
5   Tongue depressors
1   Reflex hammer
1   Hat pin
2   Pairs sterile disposable gloves, large
2   Universal glass containers (for thermal sensation testing)
1   Tape measure

Sterilised Thoracocentesis Equipment

1    $23\frac{1}{2} \times 19\frac{1}{2}$ in. (60 × 50 cm) fenestrated drape
8    $3\frac{1}{2} \times 3\frac{1}{2}$ in. (9 × 9 cm) gauze dressings
2   Pairs surgical dressing forceps
1   90 × 1.2 mm (18G) needle for exploratory puncture
2   Suture needles
1   Scalpel
1   Trocar drain
1   Plastic bag with connector for collecting the drained liquid

1	Pair sterile disposable gloves, large
1	Rectangular cup for detergent
1	Rectangular cup for disinfecting agents
4	Pads
2	10 ml syringes
1	38 × 1.2 mm (18G) needle for drug aspiration
1	15 × 0.5 mm (25G) needle for skin weal
1	38 × 0.8 mm (21G) needle for local anaesthesia
1	Dual suction valve
1	Coil of adhesive bandage 75 mm wide
1	10 ml 1% Xylocaine, attached outside pack in clear PVC wrapping
2	3/0 black silk sutures with needles
2	3/0 plain catgut sutures with needles
25	Sterile gauze swabs (5 packets of 5)
25	Sterile cotton wool balls (5 packets of 5)
2	10 ml Savlon sachets (or chlorhexidine 1% solution)

Individual Packs of Equipment

Pack 1: Medical Equipment to be Held Within a Diving Bell

1	Tourniquet (large)
1	Mouth-to-mouth resuscitator (Brook airway professional model)
1	Pair 7 in. (12.5 cm) Mayo scissors
2	Dressings (Shell or Field), large
5	Individually wrapped sterile adhesive dressings
1	Roll 1 in. (2.5 cm) adhesive tape (Elastoplast)
6	Safety pins, various sizes

Pack 2: Medical Equipment to be held Within a Deck Compression Chamber

2	Tourniquets (large)
2	Mouth-to-mouth resuscitators (Brook airway professional model)
1	Disposable oropharyngeal airway size 3
1	Disposable oropharyngeal airway size 4
1	Foot-operated sucker
1	Fine endotracheal sucker
1	Yankauer sucker (wide bore)
1	Mouth gag
1	Pair 7 in. (12.5 cm) Mayo scissors
1	Pair Spencer Wells artery forceps (12 cm or 5 in.)
1	Pair Spencer Wells artery forceps (18 cm or 7 in.)
2	Dressings (Shell or Field), large
1	Drip stand or hook
1	Roll 1 in. (2.5 cm) adhesive tape (Elastoplast)

Pack 3: Respiratory and Resuscitation Equipment

1	Laerdal resuscitator bag with a 100% oxygen fitting and with fitting to BIBS
1	Laerdal pocket mask
1	†Laryngoscope with batteries
1	†No. 9 endotracheal tube
1	†No. 9.5 endotracheal tube
1	†Oesophageal obturator airway
1	Disposable oropharyngeal airway size 3
1	Disposable oropharyngeal airway size 4
1	Mouth-to-mouth resuscitator (Brook airway professional model)
1	Pair 7 in. (12.5 cm) Mayo scissors
1	Foot-operated sucker
2	Fine endotracheal suckers
1	Yankauer sucker (wide bore)
1	Mouth gag
1	1 in. (2.5 cm) roll gauze tape
1	Tube lubricating jelly
1	Pair 5 in. (12 cm) Spencer Wells artery forceps
1	20 ml syringe

Pack 4: Intravenous Cut-Down, Suturing and Arrest of Haemorrhage Equipment

1	Tourniquet (large)
3	Pairs Spencer Wells artery forceps (12 cm or 5 in.)
1	Pair Spencer Wells artery forceps (18 cm or 7 in.)
1	Sterilised 'cut-down' kit containing:

  1 disposable scalpel
  2 scalpel blades
  1 pair pointed scissors
  1 pair toothed dissecting forceps
  1 pair fine-toothed dissecting forceps
  2 pairs mosquito forceps
  1 aneurysm needle
  1 small retractor
  1 pair needle holders
  2 × 2/0 catgut plain on atraumatic needles ⎫ (in packs
  2 × 0   catgut plain on atraumatic needles ⎬ attached to
  4 × 3/0 black silk on atraumatic needles ⎭ exterior)

25	Sterile gauze swabs (5 packets of 5)
25	Sterile cotton wool balls (5 packets of 5)
2	10 ml 1% Xylocaine
3	10 ml Savlon sachets (or chlorhexidine 1% solution)

---

†These items only to be used by an attendant specifically trained in intubation technique

Pack 5: Intravenous Infusion Equipment, All Drugs Including Resuscitation Drugs

Should be labelled 'Normally to be opened only on the advice of a doctor'

3	Intravenous giving sets with long drip chambers (e.g. Baxter)
2	20 ml syringes
2	5 ml syringes
2	2 ml syringes
5	No. 21 1½ in. (3.5 cm) hypodermic needles
5	No. 25 1 in. (2.5 cm) hypodermic needles
4	Medicut cannulae size 16
4	Medicut cannulae size 18
2	Butterfly infusion sets 19G
4	Plastic bottle holders
1	Pair 12 cm (5 in.) Spencer Wells artery forceps
1	Pair 18 cm (7 in.) Spencer Wells artery forceps
2	Sequestrene bottles
4	Plain blood bottles
20	Sealed alcohol swabs for cleaning skin
1	Short arm splint (board for i.v.)
2	3 in. crepe bandages (7.5 cm)
2	1 in. (2.5 cm) rayon porous synthetic adhesive tape
20	Sterile gauze swabs (4 packets of 5)
20	Sterile cotton wool balls (4 packets of 5)
1	10 ml 1% Xylocaine
1	10 ml Savlon sachet (or chlorhexidine 1% solution)
2	500 ml bottle dextran 70 in saline
2	1 l bottles dextrose saline
4	500 ml bottles normal saline
1	250 ml mannitol 10%
1	5 ml heparin injections 5000 units/ml
4	Diazepam injections 10 mg in 2 ml
5	Diazepam tablets 5 mg
5	2 ml dexamethasone injections 4 mg/ml
20	Dexamethasone tablets 2 mg
10	Injections soluble hydrocortisone 100 mg (i.v. or i.m.)
2	2 ml frusemide injections 10 mg/ml
2	2 ml prochlorperazine injections 12.5 mg/ml
2	1 ml chlorpheniramine injections 10 mg/ml
2	10 ml adrenaline injections 1:10 000
2	10 ml calcium gluconate injections 10%
2	Atropine injections 0.6 mg/ml
4	50 ml sodium bicarbonate 8.4% solution (1 m equiv./ml)
25	Cinnarizine tablets
1	Bottle soluble dextrose tablets
25	Soluble aspirin tablets
1	50 g silver sulphadiazine cream 1%
3	Morphine sulphate injections 15 mg in 2 ml to be included with this pack, but only if they can be stored separately in a locked cabinet within a locked cupboard, listed in the Controlled Drugs Register and regularly accounted for

Pack 6: Diagnostic Equipment

1	Pencil torch with batteries
1	Thermocouple thermometer or means of measuring temperature
1	Stethoscope
1	Aneroid sphygmomanometer with a hole drilled in the outer case
1	Auriscope with spare batteries and ophthalmic eyepiece
1	Tuning fork 128 Hz
1	Tuning fork 512 Hz
1	Bottle urine testing strips (Haemocombistix)
5	Tongue depressors
1	Reflex hammer
1	Hat pin
2	Pairs sterile disposable gloves, large
2	Universal glass containers (for thermal sensation testing)
1	Tape measure

Pack 7: Sterile Thoracocentesis 'Chest Drain' Equipment

Should be labelled 'Normally to be opened only on the advice of a doctor'

1	$23\frac{1}{2} \times 19\frac{1}{2}$ in. (60 × 50 cm) fenestrated drape
8	$3\frac{1}{2} \times 3\frac{1}{2}$ in. (9 × 9 cm) gauze dressings
2	Pairs surgical dressing forceps
1	90 × 1.2 mm (18G) needle for exploratory puncture
2	Suture needles
1	Scalpel
1	Trocar drain
1	Plastic bag with connector for collecting the drained liquid
1	Pair sterile disposable gloves, large
1	Rectangular cup for detergent
1	Rectangular cup for disinfecting agents
4	Pads
2	10 ml syringes
1	38 × 1.2 mm (18G) needle for drug aspiration
1	15 × 0.5 mm (25G) Needle for skin weal
1	38 × 0.8 mm (21G) needle for local anaesthesia
1	Dual suction valve (Heimlich)
1	Roll adhesive bandage 75 mm wide
2	3/0 black silk sutures with needles
2	3/0 plain catgut sutures with needles
25	Sterile gauze swabs (5 packets of 5)
25	Sterile cotton wool balls (5 packets of 5)
2	10 ml Savlon sachets (or chlorhexidine 1% solution)
1	10 ml 1% Xylocaine, attached outside pack in clear PVC wrapping

Pack 8: Urinary Catheterisation Equipment

Should be labelled 'Normally to be opened only on the advice of a doctor'

2	Small dressing bowls
1	Self-retaining Foley type catheter SR size 16 (pre-sterilised)
1	Self-retaining Foley type catheter SR size 18 (pre-sterilised)
4	Catheter spigots
2	20 ml amps. sterile water
2	Sterile urinary drainage bags
2	20 ml syringes
5	Pairs sterile disposable gloves, large
2	Tubes sterile urethral anaesthetic gel and nozzle
5	Sterile gauze swabs (1 packet of 5)
5	Sterile cotton wool balls (1 packet of 5)
2	10 ml Savlon sachets (or chlorhexidine 1% solution)

Pack 9: Sundry First-Aid Equipment and Dressings

1	Roll 1 in. (2.5 cm) adhesive tape (Elastoplast)
2	Sterile standard dressing packs, large
2	Sterile standard dressing packs, medium
2	Sterile standard dressing packs, small
6	Triangular bandages
6	Safety pins, various sizes
10	Adhesive dressings, various sizes
1	Tube cetrimide 0.5% cream
25	Sterile cotton wool balls (5 packets of 5)
25	Sterile gauze swabs (5 packets of 5)
2	10 ml Savlon sachets (or chlorhexidine 1% solution)

Appendix 4

Medical Equipment for Use in a Major Disaster

No. 3 airways	3
No. 4 airways	3
Haemaccel	40 units
Dextran 70	20 units
Saline 0.9%	40 units
Sodium bicarbonate 4.2%	6 units
Mannitol 20%	4 units
Hartmann's solution	20 units
Recipient sets A100 S61A	30
Air inlet S63	30
Venflon 14G S34	20
Venflon 18G S34	20
Polythene bags (small)	30
Polythene bags (medium)	30
Polythene bags (large; body bags)	12
Space blankets	20
Large mine dressings No. 15	24
Medium mine dressings No. 14	24
Small mine dressings No. 13	12
Patient evacuation sheets	3

Addresses of Committees and Societies Connected with Diving

1. E.U.B.S.   European Undersea Biomedical Society,
               Dr. T. Shields, North Sea Hyperbaric Centre,
               Howe Moss Drive, Dyce Aberdeen, AB2 0GL, Scotland

2. U.M.S.   Undersea Medical Society,
               9650 Rockville Pike, Bethesda, Maryland 20014, USA

3. D.M.A.C.   The Diving Medical Advisory Committee,
               28/30 Little Russell Street, London WC1A 2HN, England

4. A.O.D.C.   Association of Offshore Diving Contractors,
               28/30 Little Russell Street, London WC1A 2HN, England

5. E.D.T.C.   European Diving Technology Committee,
               Surg. Cdr. J.J.F. Liekens, c/o Belgische Geologische Dienst,
               1040 Brussels, Jennerstraat 13, Belgium

6. S.U.T.   Society of Underwater Technology,
               1 Birdcage Walk, London SW1H 9JJ, England

7. M.R.C.   Medical Research Council Decompression Sickness Panel,
               20 Park Crescent, London W1, England

8. A.D.C.   Association of Diving Contractors,
               1799 Stumpf Boulevard, Bldg. 7, Suite 4, Gretna La., 70053,
               USA

Appendix 6

Training Programmes for Offshore Rig Medics and First-Aiders

From the Draft Guidance Notes to the Proposed Offshore Installations and Pipeline Works (First-Aid) Regulations 1986

Training of Offshore Medics

25. The aim of training is, accordingly, to fit candidates for posts as offshore medics by providing them with the basic medical and nursing knowledge and practical skills to enable them:

   (a)   to communicate effectively with shore-based medical services and to apply such care or treatment as they direct;

   (b)   to co-operate with and provide treatment in accordance with the directions of a medical practitioner in circumstances where it is not practicable or necessary for the latter to attend a patient offshore;

   (c)   to give appropriate treatment to all persons suffering from illness or injury offshore where such illness or injury does not require skilled medical attention or until skilled medical attention becomes available and to equip them to:

   (i)   take a concise, accurate history of the patient's symptoms;

   (ii)   perform a clinical examination;

   (iii)   establish basic information regarding the patient's physical state, e.g. pulse, temperature, respiration, blood pressure;

   (iv)   have knowledge of the availability of other medical services, mobile or shore-based;

   (v)   transmit relevant medical information to a shore-based medical service;

   (vi)   understand and comply with the medical advice and directions of a medical practitioner when received;

   (vii)   give basic bedside care to sick and injured personnel;

   (viii) undertake treatment for minor ailments and injuries, and supervise the continuation of such treatment;

   (ix)   initiate appropriate first-aid measures in cases of serious accident or illness;

   (x)   apply appropriate resuscitative measures and initial treatment in cases of unconsciousness, immersion and hypothermia;

   (xi)   exceptionally, in an emergency, to carry out procedures such as: (a) intravenous therapy and urinary bladder catheterisation (where practicable, only after consultation with and on the directions of a suitably qualified medical practitioner); and (b) endotracheal intubation;

   (xii)   initiate procedures designed to stabilise a patient's medical condition and maintain vital functions;

   (xiii) prepare patients for transport ashore by air or sea, give appropriate information to the cabin crew regarding the patient's condition and, if necessary, be prepared to accompany the patient ashore;

   (xiv) recognise common infectious conditions and implement appropriate methods of isolation and treatment;

(xv)   recognise common dental conditions, including indications for the emergency use of analgesics;

(xvi)   recognise common psychological and psychiatric conditions;

(xvii)   know the effects and side-effects of available drugs and the indications and contra-indications for their use in treatment;

(xviii)   be aware of the hazards of diving and understand the correct procedures for treating medical conditions associated with diving;

(d)   maintain adequate medical records of illness and injury, and be able to write brief reports and letters of referral about patients;

(e)   be capable of giving simple advice to offshore personnel regarding their health problems and of indicating methods of improving general health;

(f)   understand hygiene requirements offshore and be able to recommend improvements where required;

(g)   know the occupational and toxicological hazards offshore and, so far as possible and in conjunction with other personnel, to give advice as to how these hazards may be minimised;

(h)   maintain the sick bay, its equipment and medical stores, order supplies and keep records of materials and drug usage;

(i)   be familiar with his or her role in any plan designed to cope with a major offshore emergency or disaster;

(j)   know the statutory requirements and responsibilities associated with the provision of offshore medical services, and be able to give advice on how to comply with such requirements.

26.   Offshore medics should study and be examined in the subjects required for the offshore first-aider's training course (see para 33). In addition, the course of instruction for offshore medics should include the following subjects:

(a)   Hypothermia, hyperthermia

(b)   Airway maintenance, artificial ventilation

(c)   Intravenous infusions

(d)   Urinary bladder catheterisation

(e)   Endotracheal intubation

(f)   Communicable (including sexually transmitted) diseases and infectious conditions

(g)   Eye conditions

(h)   Ear conditions

(i)   Skin conditions

(j)   Dental conditions

(k)   Hyperbaric environment

(l)   Decompression and its complications

(m)   Individual clinical instruction as required

(n)   Emergency medical services

(p)   Communications, installation/barge to shore

(q)   Offshore occupational hazards and their prevention

(r)   Offshore hygiene requirements

(s)   Psychiatric conditions

(t)   Background to the offshore industry and offshore activities

(u)   Standing orders and disaster plans

(v)   Use and administration of drugs

(*w*)   Stores and equipment

(*x*)   Statutory requirements

(*y*)   Keeping of detailed records.

27.   The course, including examinations, should normally take at least four full weeks.

28.   Offshore Medic Certificates will be valid for three years only. A refresher course, followed by re-examination, will be required before re-certification.

Refresher Courses

29.   Refresher courses for offshore medics should be full time (i.e. occupying complete working days) and should last for at least two weeks. Courses should ensure considerable practical re-training, as well as providing a summary of advances in knowledge and a review of relevant practical offshore experience. They should include the following subjects:

(*a*)   Acute medical and surgical emergencies

(*b*)   Immersion

(*c*)   Hypothermia, hyperthermia

(*d*)   Unconsciousness

(*e*)   Shock, haemorrhage

(*f*)   Hyperbaric medicine

(*g*)   Minor ailments

(*h*)   Revision of techniques and procedures

(*i*)   Medical services and communications

(*j*)   Transport of patients

(*k*)   Drugs and equipment

(*l*)   Records

(*m*)   Statutory requirements

(*n*)   Recent developments

Instructors

30.   The training should be given by at least two persons drawn from categories (a)–(d) below, at least one of whom should be a medical practitioner with knowledge and experience of basic health care and working conditions offshore:

(*a*)   Medical practitioners, or nurses, with knowledge and experience of basic health care and working conditions offshore;

(*b*)   Graduate lecturers or qualified teachers who hold a current Offshore First-aid Certificate and who have practical experience of first-aid offshore;

(*c*)   Offshore medics who hold a certificate which is issued by an organisation whose training of lay first-aid instructors is acceptable to the Secretary of State and which shows that they are competent to teach;

(*d*)   Instructors with practical experience of first-aid offshore who hold a current Offshore First-aid Certificate and a certificate issued by an organisation whose training of lay first-aid instructors is acceptable to the Secretary of State and which shows that they are competent to teach.

Examinations

31. Examinations should be conducted by two qualified instructors (see para 30 above), at least one of whom should be a medical practitioner with knowledge and experience of basic health care and working conditions offshore. At least one examiner should be drawn from outside the organisation or company running the course. The examination should cover both theory and practice.

Training of Offshore First-Aiders

General Responsibilities of Offshore First-Aiders

32. The main responsibilities of the offshore first-aider are as follows:

(a) To provide trained escorts for sick or injured persons being evacuated ashore;

(b) To assist in the management of serious incidents involving multiple casualties;

(c) To provide general support to the offshore medic.

On certain smaller installations which do not require a medic to be available, a designated offshore first-aider will be in charge of the sick bay. In such circumstances, the offshore first-aider should be able to communicate effectively with shore-based medical services and, if necessary, to act on the directions of a supervising medical practitioner.

Training

33. Training courses in offshore first-aid, including examinations, should normally last at least five days or the equivalent. The following subjects should be included in the syllabus:

(a) Resuscitation

(b) Control of bleeding

(c) Management of unconscious patient

(d) Treatment of shock

(e) Treatment of hypothermia

(f) Treatment of immersion

(g) Recognition and treatment of minor illness

(h) Poisons

(i) Treatment of injuries

(j) Treatment of burns and scalds

(k) Personal hygiene in dealing with wounds

(l) Dressing and immobilisation of injured parts

(m) Re-dressing of wounds and other follow-up treatment which can be undertaken by offshore first-aiders

(n) Transport of sick and injured patients (including understanding of the difficulties of transport by helicopter and the management of patients during flight)

(p) Contents of first-aid boxes and their uses

(q) Communication and delegation in an emergency

(r) Simple record keeping

34. Offshore First-aid Certificates will be valid for 3 years only. A refresher course, followed by re-examination, will be required before re-certification.

Refresher Courses

35.   Refresher courses for offshore first-aiders should be not less than two days in length and should include:

(*a*)   A demonstration of emergency first-aid procedures;

(*b*)   A revision and updating of techniques and procedures and, where appropriate, a demonstration of new techniques and procedures.

Instructors

36.   The training should be given by persons drawn from the categories listed in para 30.

Examination

37.   Offshore first-aid examinations should be conducted by two qualified instructors (see para 30), at least one of whom should be a medical practitioner, or a nurse, with knowledge and experience of basic health care and working conditions offshore, or a qualified offshore medic (i.e. one who holds an Offshore Medic Certificate). The examination should cover both theory and practice. Every candidate should be required to demonstrate proficiency in resuscitation, control of bleeding and management of the unconscious patient.

Format for Routine Offshore Hygiene Inspections
From the UKOOA Environmental Health Guidelines for Offshore Installations

Routine Environmental Health Report

Date: **Reference**

OIM/OIC
Installation   Caterers
Location   Number of employees
Strength   Camp boss
Number of beds   Installation medical staff

Part One: Food Hygiene and Catering Facilities

No.	Item	Observations
1.	Structure	
2.	Floors	
3.	Equipment	
4.	Working surfaces	
5.	Lighting	
6.	Ventilation	
7.	Drainage	
8.	Waste disposal	
9.	Water supply	
10.	First aid	
11.	Handwashing facilities	
12.	Notices	
13.	Staff sanitary accommodation	
14.	Storage of outdoor clothing	
15.	Cleaning materials	
16.	Dry goods storage	
17.	Fruit and vegetable storage	
18.	Frozen food storage	
19.	Defrosting arrangements	
20.	Milk and ice-cream	
21.	Slicing machines Butchery equipment	
22.	Storage of cooked meats Storage of prepared foods	

23. Food presentation and display
24. Food handling
25. Medical examination of food handlers and ancillary staff
26. Personal hygiene — food handlers, and ancillary staff
27. Washing up arrangements
28. ⎫
29. ⎬ Spare
30. ⎪
31. ⎭

Part Two: Accommodation Areas

32. Cabins
33. Sanitary accommodation
34. Laundry facilities
35. Recreation areas
36. Beverage making areas
37. Heating
38. Artificial ventilation
39. Natural ventilation
40. Lighting cabins
41. Lighting common parts
42. ⎫
43. ⎬ Spare
44. ⎭

General Remarks

Part Three: Summary of Defects

Serial   Recommendations

Defects Previously Reported

Serial	Date	Remedied Yes/No	Serial	Date	Remedied Yes/No

Distribution (as directed by the operator's policy)
. . . . Installation Medical Staff

Quarterly Environmental Health Report

Date: Reference

OIM/OIC
Installation   Caterers
Location   Number of employees
Strength   Camp boss
Number of beds   Installation medical staff

Part One: Summary of Defects

Serial   Observations

General Remarks:

Distribution (as directed by the operator's policy)

Signed: ....
Date ....

Part Two: Food Hygiene and Catering Facilities

Serial	Item	Observations
1.	Structure Repair Decoration Cleanliness	
2.	Floors Repair Cleanliness	
3.	Equipment Cleanliness Condition	

4.	Working surfaces Repair Cleanliness	

5.	Lighting Standard Safety	

6.	Ventilation Efficiency Cleanliness Repair	

7.	Drainage Fittings Repair Cleanliness	

8.	Waste disposal Storage Collection Bulk storage and disposal	

9.	Water supply Date last sampled Result of bacteriological examination Chemical sampling carried out Yes/No	

10.	First aid Location of box Contents Person in charge	

11.	Handwashing facilities Hot and cold water supply Soap Nailbrushes Hand drying facilities Cleanliness	

12.	Notices Displayed Required Yes/No Handwashing No smoking	

13.	Staff sanitary accommodation Location Repair Cleanliness	

14.	Outdoor clothing
	Kept in food rooms
	Suitable storage provided

15.	Cleaning materials
	Where stored
	Detergents
	Sterilising agents

16.	Dry goods storage
	Cleanliness
	Fittings
	Repair
	Ventilation
	Capacity
	Infestations
	Packaging

17.	Fruit and vegetable storage
	Location
	Cleanliness
	Fittings
	Ventilation
	Infestations
	Capacity
	Protection

18.	Frozen food storage
	Location
	Cleanliness
	Shelving
	Packaging
	Temperature control
	Capacity
	Safety
	Repair

19.	Defrosting arrangements
	Equipment
	Repair
	Cleanliness
	Location
	Temperature control

20.	Milk and ice-cream
	Storage
	Dispensing
	Equipment
	Cleaning and sterilisation
	Temperature control

21.	Slicing machines and butchery equipment
	Repair
	Cleanliness
	Sterilising procedures
	Safety

22.	Storage and protection of cooked meats and prepared foods
	Storage
	Cleanliness
	Protection
	Temperature control
	Location

23.	Food presentation and display
	Equipment
	Repair
	Protection
	Temperature control

24.	Food handling
	Protective clothing
	Hands
	Skin
	Hair

25.	Medical examination of food handlers and ancillary staff
	State
	Pre-employment examination not done (Name)

26.	Personal hygiene — food handlers and ancillary staff

27.	Washing up arrangements

28.	Spare

29.	Spare

30.	Spare

31.	Spare

Part Three: Living Accommodation

32.	Cabins
	Repair
	Cleanliness
	Overcrowding
	Lighting
	Ventilation
	Infestations

33.	Sanitary accommodation
	Fittings
	Repair
	Cleanliness
	Drainage
	Lighting
	Heating
	Ventilation
	Scale

34.	Laundry facilities
	Equipment
	Cleanliness
	Drainage
	Lighting
	Ventilation

35.	Recreation areas
	Description
	Cleanliness
	Heating
	Ventilation
	Lighting
	Scale
	Other observations

36.	Beverage making areas
	Location
	Cleanliness
	Fittings

37.	Heating and ventilation systems
	Air changes
	Temperatures
	Humidity
	Cleanliness of ducting
	Repair

38.	Artifical ventilation
	Type of plant
	Condition
	Cleanliness

39.	Natural ventilation
	Type
	Condition

40.	Lighting cabins
	Standard
	Repair
	Safety

41.	Lighting common parts
	Standard
	Repair
	Safety

42.	Drinking water
	Source of supply
	Number of points
	Notices
	Result of last bacteriological examination
	Chemical sampling carried out Yes/No

Appendix 8

Health and Safety; Draft, The Offshore Installations and Pipeline Works (First-Aid) Regulations 1986

The following are the main points from the above proposed regulations, which are likely to come into effect before 31 December 1986.

Citation

The Regulations will be called The Offshore Installations and Pipeline Works (First-Aid) Regulations 1986.

Interpretation

The Regulations are made under the Health and Safety at Work Act 1974. The meaning of first-aid is specified and offshore installation is defined as an offshore installation within the meaning of Article 4(2) of the 1977 order (application outside Great Britain) of the Health and Safety at Work Act.

The person in control is defined as:

1. The installation manager or the person made responsible by the owner for matters of health and safety or

2. The owner, and

3. Every person who is a concession owner.

Similarly, the owner of a pipeline is also defined, and the owner of an installation is defined as in Section 12 of the Mineral Workings (Offshore Installations) Act 1971. Finally, the employer of any persons engaged in any activity in connection with an offshore installation may be held responsible as 'the person in control'.

Extension of These Regulations Outside Great Britain

The Regulations will apply to any premises and activities covered by Sections 1–59 and 80–82 of the Health and Safety at Work Act by virtue of the 1977 order extending that act offshore.

Extension of Meaning of 'Work' and 'At Work'

The new regulation applies to anyone on any installation covered by the new regulations whether they are at work or not.

Duty of Person in Control

1. The person in control must ensure that all necessary equipment, facilities, medications, and suitably trained persons are provided to render first-aid and treatment under the direction of a doctor who may or may not be on the installation.

2.   He must also ensure that the medics are supervised by a qualified medical practitioner and that the advice or presence of a suitably qualified medical practitioner is available at all times.

3.   He must also ensure that all the persons at work on the installation are informed of the arrangements which have been made.

4.   The Regulations specify the training required of offshore medics and first-aiders.

5.   There will be a 2-year period of grace between the coming into effect of the Regulations and the requirement for medics to meet the training requirements imposed by the Regulations.

6.   The medically trained persons who may receive training as medics under the new Regulations are defined as a registered nurse or the holder of a certificate of competency issued within the previous 3 years by the St. John Ambulance Association of the Order of St. John or the St. Andrew's Ambulance Association or the British Red Cross Society. In addition such persons must have received adequate training in the use of mechanical artificial respiration equipment.

7.   The Regulations prescribe the siting and construction of sickbays but will not require sickbays in current use on installations to be modified as long as they have the following features:

   (i)   Interior surfaces which can be kept clean easily
   (ii)   A bath accessible from three sides
   (iii)   a water closet and wash hand-basin
   (iv)   a supply of sufficient hot and cold water for the bath and wash basin.

Exceptions to the Regulations

The Regulations do not apply to any vessel which is subject to the Merchant Shipping (Medical Scales) Regulations 1974 or which is not an offshore installation by definition.

Defence in Proceedings for Contravening These Regulations

Anyone who is alleged to have contravened the Regulations may provide a satisfactory defence if he can show that he took all reasonable precautions and exercised all due diligence to prevent the alleged offence.

Power to Grant Exemptions

The Secretary of State for Energy will be able to grant exemption to any or all of the requirements of the Regulations as long as he is satisfied that the health, safety and welfare of the persons on the installation will not be prejudiced.

Amendment and Revocations

The Regulations replace parts of the Health and Safety (First-Aid) Regulations 1981 and the Offshore Installations (Operational Safety, Health and Welfare) Regulations 1976 and The Offshore Installations (Life Saving Appliances) Regulations 1977.

The Draft Approved Code of Practice

The Regulations also have a Code of Practice which expands and clarifies the regulations themselves. It explains that an offshore first-aider is any person who holds a current offshore first-aid certificate issued by a body approved by the Secretary of State for Energy to train, examine and certify such first-aiders. Similarly offshore medics.

   It defines 'regularly at work at one time' as those numbers normally working on the installation. Such an expression does not cover the occasional and short-term fluctuation in the normal numbers. The approved Code of Practice goes on to emphasize that medics will not be acceptable unless they have undergone the training prescribed in the document and obtained the necessary qualifications, though this part of the regulations will not be enforced for 2 years after they come into effect.

The Code of Practice then goes on to describe the sickbays which must be provided on all normally manned offshore installations. The sickbay must be clearly identified, be in charge of a medic or first-aider, be available at all times and not used for any other purpose, be locked at all times when not in use and contain suitable furniture, medications and equipment as, for example, defined in the Guidance Notes. It must also have effective, direct two-way communication with onshore medical services. It is also emphasized that there shall always be a medic or first-aider on call.

As far as the layout and siting of sickbays is concerned, the Code of Practice specifies that no major changes will be required to current sickbays, as long as they conform with the minimum requirements. The sickbays on new installations will, however, require effective mechanical ventilation, a minimum temperature of 20°C, effective lighting and emergency lighting, and adequate electrical sockets carrying a supply of 220–240 volts. They will have to have stainless steel sinks with adjacent working surfaces and with a supply of hot and cold water and drinking water. Either in, or immediately adjacent, there will need to be flush toilets for the exclusive use of the sickbay, a bath approachable from three sides and an emergency full flush shower. There will need to be adequate working surfaces of an impervious nature and easy to clean and suitable arrangements for waste disposal. The floor of the room will need to be of an impervious, non-slip material with corners and angles between floors and walls rounded. There will need to be a drain in the floor and all walls, doors, door frames and windows should have washable, hygienic finishes. The size of the sickbay is not specified, but must take into account the number of people likely to be regularly at work and the furniture and equipment it will need to contain. It is also emphasized that the sickbay may need to accommodate an ill or injured person for up to 48 hours.

The Code of Practice emphasizes the importance of the appropriate siting of the sickbay, in particular that it should be within easy access of the helideck and survival craft and that the doors of the sickbay should be wide enough to allow easy access. It also specifies that lifts which may be used to take a patient from the sickbay to the helipad must be large enough to accommodate a stretcher.

It specifies that a large area adjacent to the sickbay should be made available for conversion into a casualty clearing area in an emergency. This area must have effective communication with the sickbay.

The Code of Practice emphasizes that the sickbay must not be used as quarters for the medic or anyone else and the medic's quarters should be adjacent or within close reach of the sickbay with effective communication between them.

The Code of Practice specifies the first-aid kits which must be kept available for use in an emergency and states that appropriate first-aid kits must be kept on unmanned installations whenever persons are at work on such installations.

Numbers and Types of 'Suitable Persons'

The Code of Practice specifies the number of offshore first-aiders and medics which are required on installations in accordance with their size as follows:

Number of people at work*	Number of offshore first-aiders	Number of offshore medics
Up to 25	2	–
26 to 50	3	1
51 to 100	5	1
101–150	7	1
151–200	9	1
201 and above	Additional personnel, if required, to ensure reasonable access by all offshore workers	

*In determining whether there is a need for a medic, the number of people likely to be *regularly* at work at one time (see para 3) should be considered.

The Code of Practice specifically excludes the installations of the southern gas fields, where a medic is only required when the number of people regularly at work exceeds 50.

The Code of Practice specifically requires that a fully registered medical practitioner with knowledge and experience of conditions offshore shall always be available to provide assistance to the medic or first-aiders or to fly out to the rig if required.

Arrangements During the Construction and Dismantling of Offshore Installations

The Regulations cover any barges or other installations operating within 500 m of an offshore installation. During the construction and dismantling of an offshore installation, persons at work on it must have pedestrian access to the sickbay. The Code of Practice specifies that antihypothermia bags and a mechanical resuscitation device must always be provided along with a box containing a sufficient quantity of first-aid materials. Stretchers for transferring a sick or injured person to the sickbay must always be kept available, and the provision of medics and first-aiders and the liaison arrangements with doctors apply as if they were any other offshore installation.

Duty of Person in Control to Provide Information

The Code of Practice specifies that the person in control shall inform all workers of all medical arrangements that have been made, shall ensure that medics and offshore first-aiders are easily identifiable and shall post appropriate notices indicating the locations of the medics and first-aiders. In addition it is necessary to post in the sick bay, the radio room and the OIM's office the written instructions regarding arrangements made for liaison with medical practitioners. All notices must be provided in languages appropriate to the personnel on board.

Extract from Norwegian Regulations Regarding Medical Facilities on Offshore Installations: Royal Decree, 25 November, 1977, Relating to Hygiene, Medical Equipment and Medicines, etc., on Installations for Production, etc., of Submarine Petroleum Resources, etc.

Chapter III — Medical examination, first aid equipment, medical supplies and medicines, and contingency plans for cases of illness or injury

Section 15 (Medical examination)

All personnel who are to work on such installations as mentioned in Section 2 above shall undergo such medical examination as required at any time by the Ministry of Social Affairs.

Personnel who are preparing and serving food may have to undergo more detailed medical examination. Persons suffering from contagious diseases or who are carriers of such diseases, may be restricted in their work by the Ministry of Social Affairs or may be refused permission to work on installations offshore.

Section 16 (Nursing services)

A registered nurse shall be employed on such manned installations as mentioned in Section 2 above. Instructions shall be drawn up listing the duties and areas of responsibility of the nurse, and shall be subject to approval by the Ministry of Social Affairs.

Section 17 (Medical services and medical care)

Such installations as mentioned in Section 2 above shall arrange for an agreement with a physician who shall be professionally responsible for health services on the installation.

The licensee shall also arrange for an agreement to be concluded ensuring that a physician can be contacted at any time and can come to the installation at short notice.

It is the duty of the licensee to ensure the availability of transport for the doctor to visit the installation and for a sick or injured person to be moved to a hospital or other health care facility ashore, and to pay for the cost of such transport.

In cases of illness or injury the nurse shall have unhindered priority access to radio and other telecommunication equipment in order to communicate with the physician on duty. (cf. para 2 above)

Section 18 (Health office)

Such installations as mentioned in Section 2 shall have a health office.

On major installations the health office shall consist of one or more consulting rooms/treatment rooms, sick room(s) and work room for the nurse. The health office must be furnished and equipped in such a manner that the health personnel will be able to carry out their duties in a satisfactory manner.

The rooms must be of adequate size, and none of them shall have a floor area smaller than 15 m². Consulting rooms shall have the following equipment:

an examination/treatment couch, a work table for the nurse, a lockable medicine cupboard, a handbasin with fittings for mixing hot and cold water, emergency lighting and an alarm system.

Consulting rooms shall have emergency lighting and a power supply sufficient to permit work to continue there in emergencies.

At least one of the consulting rooms shall have a lockable cupboard for dangerous drugs, a refrigerator for proper storage of drugs which need refrigeration, a laboratory area and a permanent telephone with its own telephone number.

Consulting rooms and work rooms shall have essential office furniture and equipment and lockable filing cabinets.

The sick room(s) shall be furnished and equipped to permit short-term in-patient care, e.g. while waiting for transport. Sick rooms shall not have more than two beds each.

In connection with the sick room there must be a bathroom with shower, toilet and handbasin with fittings for mixing hot and cold water. There must also be one bath tub for the treatment of hypothermia.

The number of beds for in-patients shall be calculated in relation to the total number of persons present at the installation at any time. The beds must be placed so as to allow free access from at least three sides. The sick room shall have a wardrobe locker, a bedside table and an emergency calling system. The emergency calling system shall be connected to a permanently staffed room and to the bedroom of the nurse on duty.

On smaller installations the functions of the health office may be combined in one room of adequate size, at least 20 m². It shall be furnished and equipped as described above. A hospital bed may serve as an examination/treatment couch if it has sufficient equipment. When it is used as a treatment couch it must be placed so as to allow free access from all four sides.

The health office shall be adequately insulated against noise and have heating, ventilation and lighting in accordance with Sections 12, 13 and 14 above as well as with the regulations for living quarters, etc. of the Norwegian Petroleum Directorate.

The health office should as far as possible have access to daylight.

Health office rooms shall not be used for any other purpose.

The health office shall be situated in such a manner as to permit safe and reliable stretcher transport into and out of its rooms.

Section 19 (Medical equipment, medicines, etc.)

Installations such as mentioned in Section 2 shall have medical and nursing equipment, medicines, first aid equipment including medical resuscitation equipment, as well as instruments and other equipment for control of hygiene, in accordance with the current requirements of the Ministry of Social Affairs.

Medical resuscitation equipment and other first aid equipment shall be conveniently located and packed in such a manner that adequate first aid may be given in cases of illness or injury and during transport to hospital.

The installation shall have an adequate number of stretchers conveniently located and instantly accessible. The stretchers shall be of a design which will permit safe and reliable transport of a patient to the health office, to the helicopter or to other means of transportation to shore. The Ministry may issue further instructions concerning the quality of stretchers.

Section 20 (Storage and supervision of medicines)

Medicines should be ordered from one permanent source of supply and should be issued on prescription or by a written purchase order signed and dated by the physician.

The nurse is responsible for the proper storage of medicines, and shall check that supplies received from the supplier are in accordance with the prescription or purchase order before the supplies are taken into stock. A record shall be kept of all purchases of medicines.

Medicines shall be stored in lockable cupboards intended solely for this purpose. Only the nurse on duty shall hold the keys to the medicine stores.

Medical cupboards or stores shall be large enough to ensure that all medicines may be stored in an orderly manner. The health office shall have a refrigerator for the proper storage of drugs which need refrigeration.

Medicines which are labelled 'I giftskap' or 'Dangerous drugs' shall be kept in a lockable cupboard with its own, separate key.

Only medicines and items used for medical purposes as well as medicine glasses, pipettes, etc. which are used to dispense medicines may be stored in medicine cupboards.

Medicines shall be stored in the container in which they are issued from the chemist. Transfer to other bulk containers is not permitted.

The tidiness and cleanliness of the medical cupboard is the responsibility of the nurse at all times.

Medicines may only be dispensed by persons who have been authorised to do so, cf. Instructions concerning the duties and areas of responsibility of nurses employed on installations for production, etc. of submarine petroleum resources, approved by the Ministry of Social Affairs. Such authority may only in exceptional cases be given to persons who are not registered nurses.

The dispensing of medicines shall be done in a manner which ensures that medicines are given out to the person they are intended for. In general medicines should be dispensed in amounts which correspond to a single dose. If larger quantities are dispensed they shall be given out in a suitable container with the name of the medicine and instructions for its use clearly written on the container. Records shall be kept of all issue of medicines.

Medicines shall be transported with proper care to ensure that they do not go astray or in any way cause harm or risk. During transport the containers should be locked or sealed if possible.

Supervision of the storage, dispensing and use of medicines is the responsibility of the physician, cf. Section 18, para 1, who shall ensure that the supply of medicines is satisfactory. The medical store shall be inspected annually by a pharmacist.

Pharmacist inspectors or other inspectors appointed by the Ministry of Social Affairs shall have the right to inspect the medicine store, etc.

Appendix 10

Control of Noise and Vibration on Offshore Installations (from Offshore Installations: Guidance on Design and Construction. HMSO)

Part II Section 5

5.9 Noise and vibration

This section describes the way in which noise and vibration, as affecting human exposure, should be taken into account in the design and construction of offshore installations. It details recommended maximum levels for all areas of the installation and provides basic guidelines to be followed when designing and laying out an installation to minimise potential noise and vibration problems.

This section does not attempt to give a comprehensive design guide since each installation will clearly present particular problems, depending upon its size and function. It is important that consideration of noise and vibration should form an integral part of the platform design from the inception of the project, when, for instance, major changes in platform layout can be made, to reduce potential problems. Where necessary, specialist advice should be obtained. For acoustic design purposes all calculations should be performed in the eight octave bands centred between 63 Hz and 8 kHz (see BSI 2475). The noise rating curve numerically 5 dB less than the dBA criterion, should be used as an approximate limit for the frequency spectrum of the noise. The overriding requirement, however, is that the dBA level should be met.

Noise levels should be limited throughout the installation in order to:

(a) minimise the risk of hearing damage to personnel in work areas;
(b) ensure that warning signals are audible;
(c) allow adequate speech, telephone and radio communication;
(d) maintain working efficiency;
(e) provide an acceptable sleep and recreation environment in accommodation areas.

In a similar manner vibration levels should be limited in order to:

(a) prevent a health hazard to personnel;
(b) maintain proficiency of personnel in performing designated tasks;
(c) provide an acceptable sleep and recreation environment in accommodation areas.

5.9.1 Noise
5.9.1.1. *Standards and definitions*
5.9.1.1.1 Terminology
Interpretation of the terminology used in these recommendations should be in accordance with British Standard 661 Glossary of Acoustical Terms. All noise limits in this section are quoted as 'A' weighted sound pressure levels (dBA) with the exception of the overriding limits given in 5.9.1.2. In all cases the reference sound pressures is 20×10^{-5} N/m².
5.9.1.1.2 Application of criteria
The noise criteria should be met in full at any spatial location within a designated area to which personnel may have access, except for work areas and other areas housing noisy equipment where, for design purposes, the recommended criteria should generally apply at a minimum distance of 1 metre from

operational equipment. If personnel are normally required to work closer than a distance of 1 metre to equipment then the noise criteria should also apply at these locations.

5.9.1.2 *Criteria*

5.9.1.2.1 Maximum permissible noise levels (overriding limits)

Notwithstanding the criteria specified for the designated areas, under no operational design condition should the unprotected ear be exposed to sound pressure levels exceeding 135 dB (linear).

5.9.1.2.2 General work area noise limits

All areas other than those stated in Sections 5.9.1.2.3 and 5.9.1.2.4 should meet the general work area noise level limit of 88 dBA for a 12-hour working day. This limit is based on hearing damage risk considerations and is derived from the requirements of the Department of Employment's 'Code of Practice for Reducing the Exposure of Employed Persons to Noise'. If shift lengths are less than 12 hours then the noise limit may be increased in accordance with this code of practice, i.e. a noise limit of 90 dBA will apply for an eight-hour shift. These limits generally apply for broad band noise. Where a noise exhibits dominant tonal characteristics, then it is desirable to suppress such characteristics.

5.9.1.2.3 Specific work area noise limits

Where reliable speech, telephone or radio communication is required, or demanding mental tasks must be performed, then the noise limits for these areas should be considerably less than the limit for general work areas. Recommended noise limits for particular work areas such as control rooms, etc. are given in Table 5.3. Any tonal characteristic should be suppressed so as not to give rise to annoyance. These limits refer to background noise, including ventilation and external noise sources, but not to manually controlled operations involving inherently noisy equipment, e.g. drilling, mixing, etc. for which general work area noise limits shall apply. This does not include the radio/telecommunications room in which noisy office equipment, e.g. telex machines, should either not be installed or should be suitably quietened.

Table 5.3 Recommended noise limits for specific work areas of offshore installations

Specific work areas of offshore installations	Noise limit, dBA
Workshops	70
General stores	70
Kitchens	60
Control rooms	55
Offices	55
Laboratories	55
Radio/Communication rooms	45

5.9.1.2.4 Sleeping/recreation area noise limits

The noise limits given in Table 5.4 are recommended for those areas of living accommodation on offshore installations where satisfactory recreation, rest and sleeping conditions are required. Any tonal characteristics should be suppressed so as not to give rise to annoyance.

The limits given in Table 5.4 should be regarded as maximum acceptable noise levels for these areas. Where lower levels can be relatively easily obtained (e.g. by ventilation silencing) then it is desirable that these noise control measures should be implemented.

5.9.1.3 *Relaxation of noise limits*

5.9.1.3.1 General work area

All reasonably practicable means should be taken to comply with the specified noise levels. If the limit cannot be achieved in certain areas then these should be treated as 'restricted' and appropriate warning notices posted. Personnel entering these areas should generally be obliged to wear suitable ear protectors unless their daily unprotected noise exposure can be shown to be within the requirements of the Department of Employment's Code of Practice.

Examples of restricted areas could be as follows:

(a) Normal operational conditions: within noise control enclosures large enough to admit service personnel.

(b) Intermittent operational conditions: on the helideck when a helicopter is present.

(c) Design emergency conditions: near emergency safety relief valves.

5.9.1.3.2. All other areas
The noise limits specified for these areas should normally apply at all times although in certain circumstances this may not be practical, e.g. during helicopter movements.

Table 5.4 Recommended noise limits for sleeping/recreation areas of living accommodation on offshore installations

Sleeping/Recreation areas of living accommodation	Noise limit, dBA
Washing facilities	60
Changing rooms	60
Toilets	60
Dining rooms	55
Recreation rooms	50
Theatre/Meeting rooms	45
Television rooms	45
Sleeping areas	45
Medical rooms	45
Quiet rooms	45

Note: Noise levels in corridors should not generally be more than 5 dBA greater than the noise limits in adjoining rooms, with a maximum level of 60 dBA in any corridor.

5.9.2 Vibration
5.9.2.1 General
The vibration limits recommended in this section are derived for the acceptability of exposure of human beings to vibration (see Building Research Station Digest No. 117, May 1970, and BSI DD32, Guide to the Evaluation of Human Exposure to Whole Body Vibration), and are given as r.m.s. acceleration levels in m/sec^2.
5.9.2.2. Standards and Definitions
5.9.2.2.1 Terminology
Interpretation of the terminology used in these recommendations should be in accordance with International Standard ISO 2041, Vibration and Shock Vocabulary
5.9.2.2.2 Relevant surfaces for application of criteria
The recommended vibration limits should be met on surfaces designated as normal access for standing and sitting.
5.9.2.3 Vibration limits for human exposure
5.9.2.3.1 Exposure time
The vibration limits recommended for general work areas are based on a 12-hour working day. These limits should be taken as the design values for offshore installations. In certain circumstances some relaxation of the general work area vibration limits may be considered acceptable.
5.9.2.3.2 Frequency range
The specified criteria cover the frequency range 1–80 Hz and are not intended to be extrapolated beyond these limits.
5.9.2.3.3 Direction of vibration
Criteria are specified for both vertical and horizontal linear motion and apply separately to the resolved components of the vibration in these directions. Direction, a_z, should be taken to correspond with the foot to head axis of the human body (see BSI DD32).

Appendix 11

First-Aid Training of Divers and Diving Supervisors (AODC)

Compiled by the Diving Medical Advisory Committee, February 1983

All divers are required to be trained in first-aid to a standard appropriate to emergencies which may arise during the diving operation. Ideally, they should be trained in, and hold the kind of qualification in first-aid which can only be obtained after they have successfully completed a course which has been specifically designed to cater for the requirements of divers, including general theoretical and practical principles of first-aid.

At present, the qualifications in the United Kingdom are those of St. John, Red Cross or St. Andrew's, but each of these courses includes specialised material which is not essential first-aid for divers, and omits certain matters which are essential. The St. John Ambulance Association Certificate can no longer be issued by any organisation running its own courses, as the award of such a Certificate has to result from attendance at a course organised and run by the St. John Ambulance Association, on which the syllabus contains no less and no more than the contents of whichever of the new St. John training packages is appropriate. Therefore, such courses are obviously not suitable for divers. They are intended for onshore personnel.

In Norway, there are no comparable organisations running courses with standard universally-approved syllabi. There is a requirement for vehicle drivers, pilots, etc. to have some training in first-aid, but the extent and effective content of this, and the degree to which it is enforced seems to vary considerably over the country.

All this merely confirms the need to press forward with plans for specifically-designed courses for divers with the minimum of delay.

Following proposals put forward by the European Undersea Biomedical Society's Sub-Committee on the Training of Divers some years ago, the terms 'Medically-Trained Diver Class I' [MTD(1)] and 'Class II' [MTD(2)] were suggested, and are used in this document.

The MTD(1) course includes general first-aid, a minimum of 14 hours first-aid training, 20 hours of basic medical introduction, diving physics, physiology and diving medicine; including familiarisation with specialised medical equipment and techniques.

Worksite practical training is ideal, but in practice is extremely time-consuming and difficult to organise, particularly during an intensive course. Diving companies should however consider instituting in-house revision of first-aid skills.

There should be refresher training (shorter, concentrated periods) for all those who have successfully completed the MTD(1) course. It would be difficult to devise a syllabus for a refresher course where students have previously attended a variety of different main courses; it is suggested therefore, that refresher courses should not come into effect until one year after the MTD(1) courses have commenced.

Those divers and diving supervisors who show particular interest and natural ability should proceed to the training leading to the *qualification MTD(2)*. In any remote location at least one diver in each team and all supervisors should have achieved this standard.

At the diver's annual medical examination there is an opportunity to remind the diver how to examine a fellow diving casualty, and also to question him on his knowledge of the symptoms of decompression sickness. An alarming ignorance is frequently demonstrated during such periods of questioning. Many of those who have undergone training forget much of what they have learnt, whilst in some others this training has never been undertaken.

It is important therefore that there is refresher training which could be conducted at the original training school, or co-ordinated by the training school, or one offering equivalent training, or at some other suitable place.

The need for uniform training standards to be adopted is clear and the guidelines recommended in this document are submitted to AODC for adoption by their members and to establishments offering first aid training directed at the diving industry.

Acceptance by AODC members of these guidelines would clearly improve the present position and help to ensure that satisfactory standards of first aid training are introduced, in the interests of those who may need to use them.

MTD(1) Course

Purpose

To enable divers and diving supervisors to carry out first aid for minor incidents and to be able to take adequate action in medical emergencies until a doctor can take over treatment.

Limitations

The programme for first aid training outlined below will provide divers with sufficient knowledge and skill to administer adequate first aid under conditions where professional assistance can be obtained within about 2 hours. Where this is not the case, personnel with additional medical training (MTD(2) standard) should be present at the worksite.

Level of Training

The training is at the level indicated by the reference books:

1.   USN Diving Manual (USNDM); and
2.   WHO International Medical Guide for Ships (IMGS),

i.e. corresponding to Naval diver training and the medical training of Merchant Ships Officers.

Types of Emergency Situations Envisaged

1. *Various hyperbaric emergencies*, including:

Air embolism
Pneumothorax
Subcutaneous emphysema
Decompression sickness
Squeezes
Drowning
Hypoxia and various gas toxicities

2. *Lesions incurred during work*:

Fractures	Wounds
Dislocations	Arterial and venous bleeding
Sprains	Internal lesions
Strains	Blast and crush injuries
Burns	Electrical lesions and shock
Scalds	

3. *Various medical and surgical conditions*: infectious diseases and acute abdominal illnesses which may develop quickly in otherwise healthy persons.

Necessary Background in Anatomy, Physiology and Physics

In order that the trainee can understand the nature of various malfunctions which can occur to the body, particularly the nature of diving illnesses, a certain knowledge of anatomy and physiology is necessary. Minimal requirements should be the combined chapters on anatomy and physiology of the USNDM and IMGS (circulation, respiration, ears and sinuses are well covered in USNDM, the rest of the body is better treated in IMGS).

A knowledge of underwater physics included in the USNDM should also be a minimal requirement.

Knowledge and Skills to be Covered by the Training Programme

1. *Preparation for Emergencies*: all divers should be trained to prepare for emergencies. They should be familiar with the company emergency medical and diving procedures. This includes checking:

   A   Location and condition of first aid equipment and oxygen.
   B   Where and whom to contact for emergency services, doctor, helicopter.
   C   Location of nearest recompression chambers.

2. *Getting an unconscious or injured diver out of the water*: into a bell, onto a ship, platform, jetty, etc.

3. *Resuscitation*:

Evaluation of respiration and heart action:
  how to clear and maintain the airway (positioning — manual extraction   —
  Heimlich manoeuvre — Guerdel airway — tongue retainer).

Artificial ventilation:
  (mouth-to-mouth or nose; AMBU or Laerdal mask with air or oxygen).

External cardiac massage.

When to start and when to stop.

TRAINING FOR 2 AND 3 SHOULD BE CARRIED OUT AND REHEARSED
UNDER ACTUAL DIVING CONDITIONS.

4. *General aspects of diving emergencies*:

A   Thorough understanding of decompression sickness, arterial gas embolism
    and their preventative measures.
B   Examination of a patient and accurate reporting of his condition.
C   Ability to understand and carry out medical instructions received.
D   Complete familiarity with the company's safety and diving manuals.

5. *Diving emergencies requiring recompression*:

A   Arterial gas embolism (symptoms and objective signs: differential diagnosis
    against decompression sickness — necessity of immediate recompression —
    knowledge of the treatment tables which can be used).
B   Decompression sickness (symptoms and signs: recognition of CNS or
    cardio-pulmonary involvement — use of treatment tables according to
    symptoms and response).
C   Subcutaneous emphysema (symptoms and signs: recompression treatment
    if necessary — risks of recompression).
D   Pneumothorax (symptoms and objective signs: when to recompress and
    when not — management).

6. *Diving emergencies not necessarily requiring recompression*:

A   Hypoxia.
B   Carbon monoxide poisoning.
C   Gas expansion in ears, sinuses and gastrointestinal tract (prevention —
    symptoms — recompression treatment if necessary).

7. *Diving emergencies not requiring recompression*:

A   Drowning (resuscitation).
B   Hypothermia, immersion and cold exposure (knowledge of physiological
    mechanism — treatment [NATO STANAG 1187]).
C   Hyperthermia.
D   Squeeze (symptoms and signs: usually on treatment — prophylactic use of
    decongestants in colds — diving to be avoided — oxygen treatment of lung
    squeeze).

E   Asphyxia.
F   Hypercapnia.
G   Nitrogen narcosis.
H   Oxygen toxicity (recognition in self and others — prevention — treatment).
I   Chemical irritants.
J   High pressure nervous syndrome.
K   Rupture of the round or oval window (of the inner ear).

8. *First aid for various injuries and accidents*:

General principles:

> First aid dressing
> Treatment of severe wounds (head, body, extremities) and bleeding (arterial, venous, internal)
> Shock
> Burns; Scalds
> Crush and blast injuries
> Sprains; strains
> Dislocations
> Fractures
> Unconsciousness
> Electric shock
> Sunstroke and overheating

(IMGS, chapter 3)

9. *Oxygen treatment*: generally where cyanosis indicates a lack of oxygen.

10. *Administration of injections*: (under supervision — subcutaneous and intramuscular).

11. *Transport of patients*: various ways to move injured persons — special considerations regarding (air) transport of patients following diving.

12. *Familiarity with medical equipment*: knowledge of the contents of equipment sets for insertion of intravenous infusion, chest drains, urinary catheters and endotracheal tubes, to be able to assist a medically qualified attendant. (Note: it is not intended that a diver or supervisor should carry out any of these procedures but he *should* be able to assist an attendant qualified to do so.)

13. *Signs of death*

MTD(2) Course

First aid training to the MTD(1) standard should enable a diving supervisor or diver to examine a patient and describe his condition to a doctor, but it will not enable him to treat or nurse the patient over any extended period of time. Therefore, when divers are working under conditions where professional medical assistance cannot be provided within a period of, say, two hours, a person with additional medical training should be present at the worksite. This person must be able to work under pressure. He could be a medical technician, a nurse, a diver, or a diving supervisor who has had supplementary medical training.

The training of such persons should include, in addition to the MTD(1) training:

1. *Diagnosis*: routine history and routine physical examination to a degree of competence which should make it possible to make a diagnosis with the aid of a (radio) doctor (IMGS, chapter 5 [four pages] — possibly with additional sessions devoted to neurology).

2. *Treatment of wounds, inflammation, sprains and dislocations, fractures*: (IMGS, chapters 6–9 [42 pages]).

3. *General nursing*: includes nursing of fracture cases, nursing of unconscious or paralysed cases, the giving of subcutaneous, intramuscular and intravenous injections (IMGS, chapter 4).

4. *Special procedures*:

    A   Measurement of temperature, pulse, blood pressure and respiratory rate. Observation of skin colour, level of consciousness and general condition.
    B   Setting up an intravenous infusion to treat shock (loss of effective circulating blood volume) under (radio) guidance of a doctor.
    C   Passing a urinary catheter which may be necessary when nursing an unconscious or paralysed case.
    D   Passing a rectal tube.
    E   Passing a gastric tube.
    F   Relieving a tension pneumothorax by inserting chest tube with valve.
    G   Removal of foreign body in eye (superficial corneal).

    The procedures under B to F inclusive should only be attempted after teleconsultation with a doctor, and such communication *should* be possible at all times.

References

US Navy Diving Manual, vol. 1–2 (Navsea 0994–LP-001–9010 January 1979)
International Medical Guide for Ships. WHO, Geneva, 1967
In first aid training of divers IMGS could be replaced by any good modern textbook on first aid.
NATO STANAG 1187: Management of Acute Hypothermia

Appendix 12

In the original, pages 3–7 are red

The Diving Medical Advisory Committee

CONFIDENTIAL

AIDE-MÉMOIRE
FOR RECORDING AND TRANSMISSION
OF MEDICAL DATA TO SHORE
(1984)

This form has been designed in three parts to make it easier to use.

Part 1 (red pages) is an Aide Memoire to obtain essential information for transmission ashore in event of a medical emergency. This information will enable the onshore doctor to advise on immediate management of the casualty.

Part 2 collects more detailed information to provide a permanent record of the incident and to assist in accident analysis. Obviously in urgent cases THERE MUST BE NO DELAY in contacting medical assistance with the information in Part 1. Part 2 should be completed later.

The onshore doctor will frequently ask for some further examination to be carried out.

Part 3 provides a form for recording this information.

It is recognised that it will not be necessary to complete the form fully in most cases, and where a question (or section) is not applicable, N/A should be entered. If you are uncertain of the meaning of a question, do not attempt to answer it, but ring the question number.

Part 1

ESSENTIAL INFORMATION FOR TRANSMISSION
ASHORE IN EVENT OF AN EMERGENCY

Part 1 Section A
GENERAL INFORMATION

1   Patient surname: _____ Christian Name: _____

2   Company: _____

3   Worksite: _____

4   Date of incident: _____ Time: _____

5   Type of incident: _____

6   Is the general condition of the patient:

                            Good   [   ]

                            Fair   [   ]

                            Critical   [   ]

Part 1 Section B
INFORMATION ABOUT THE DIVE RELATED TO THE INCIDENT

(If the illness or injury is not related to diving, skip to Section E)

7   Method: Scuba   [   ]   Bell bounce   [   ]

                      Surface supplied [   ]   Saturation   [   ]

                      Wet bell   [   ]

8   Breathing mixture: Air   [   ]   Nitrox   [   ]

                      Heliox   [   ]   Trimix   [   ]

9   Job: Diver   [   ]   Other   [   ]

                      Bellman   [   ]   (Specify: _____)

10   Working depth: _____ metres

11   Bell depth (where relevant):   _____ metres

3

12 Storage depth (where relevant):   _____ metres

13 Time spent at working depth: _____ minutes

14 Decompression Table selected: _____

        Depth selected   _____ metres

        Bottom time selected   _____ minutes

        Surface interval selected   _____ hrs _____ minutes
        (repetitive dives)

15 Type of work performed: _____

    _____

    _____

    _____

16 Adverse conditions, if any: (e.g. sea state, tidal stream, temperature, fouling, disorderly ascent,
    hard work, etc.)

    _____

    _____

    _____

17 Did the incident begin: in the water [   ]   in the deck chamber [   ]

                               in the bell   [   ]   other?   [   ]

                                                           (specify: _____)

18 At the time of onset of symptoms, was the patient:

                               descending   [   ]   ascending   [   ]

                               on the bottom [   ]   on the surface   [   ]

Part 1 Section C

COMPRESSION/DECOMPRESSION INCIDENT

(If the incident is not related to a change in pressure, skip to Section E)

19 Incident during or immediately following compression   [YES]   [NO]

20 Incident during normal decompression: [YES]   [NO]

21 Incident after surfacing following normal decompression: [YES]   [NO]

    End of decompression at _____ hrs _____ mins

4

22 Incident following excursion from saturation: YES   NO

Time of outset after decompression _____ hrs _____ mins

23 Incident following blow-up/drop in pressure   YES   NO

From depth _____ metres, time _____ hrs _____ mins

To depth _____ metres, time _____ hrs _____ mins

24 In other circumstances   YES   NO

Specify: _____

_____

_____

_____

25 Onset of first symptom at: time _____ hrs _____ mins

depth _____ metres

26 Niggles   YES   NO

27 Pain in joints
(state location: _____)   YES   NO

28 Pain in muscles
(state location: _____)   YES   NO

29 Pins and needles
(state location: _____)   YES   NO

30 Patches of numbness or tingling, or altered sensation
(state location: _____)   YES   NO

31 Muscle weakness or paralysis
(state location: _____)   YES   NO

32 Difficulty in urinating   YES   NO

33 Pain in the lumbar region, around waist, or in the abdomen   YES   NO

34 Standing upright difficult or impossible   YES   NO

35 Nausea   YES   NO

36 Vomiting   YES   NO

37 Vertigo, loss of balance   YES   NO

38	Deafness, hearing problems	YES	NO
39	Speech problems	YES	NO
40	Visual problems	YES	NO
41	Drowsiness, confusion (specify: _____)	YES	NO
42	Loss of consciousness	YES	NO
43	Paleness, anxiety, sweating, collapse (specify: _____)	YES	NO
44	Cyanosis, blue skin	YES	NO
45	Breathlessness, painful breathing, chokes (specify: _____)	YES	NO
46	Blood-stained froth in airways	YES	NO
47	Respiratory distress worsening with decompression	YES	NO
48	Others (specify below:)	YES	NO

_____

_____

_____

Part 1 Section D
PREVIOUS DIVE

(If ended less than 24 hrs before the accident)

49	Method:	Scuba	☐	Bell bounce	☐
		Surface supplied	☐	Saturation	☐
		Wet bell	☐	Excursion from saturation	☐
50	Breathing mixture:	Air	☐	Nitrox	☐
		Heliox	☐	Trimix	☐

51   Depth: _____ metres

52   Bottom time (where relevant):   _____ mins

53   Table selected: _____

         Depth selected: _____ metres

         Time selected: _____ mins

6

54   Normal decompression: YES   NO

55   End of decompression:

     Day_____ / _____ Time _____ hrs _____ mins

56   If saturation, back to storage depth from last working dive:

     Day_____ / _____ Time _____ hrs _____ mins

Part 1 Section E
ACCIDENT OR ILLNESS NOT RELATED TO DECOMPRESSION

57   Nature of Accident or Illness: _____

     _____

     _____

     _____

58   Does he have difficulty or pain with breathing?   YES   NO

59   Is he bleeding?   YES   NO

60   If yes, is bleeding controlled?   YES   NO

61   State of consciousness:

          Fully alert and orientated   ☐

          Drowsy   ☐

          Confused   ☐

          Unconscious but responds to stimuli   ☐

          Unconscious and unresponsive   ☐

62   Detail symptoms: _____

     _____

     _____

     _____

63   Treatment given: _____

     _____

     _____

     _____

Part 2

ADDITIONAL INFORMATION FOR RECORD PURPOSES
**N.B. Do NOT delay transmission of Part 1 in order
to complete this part of the Form**

Part 2 Section A

GENERAL INFORMATION

1   Name of patient: _____

2   Date of birth: _____

3   Date of last medical examination: _____

4   Where medical records are held: _____

_____

5   Details of previous decompression sickness: _____

_____

_____

_____

_____

6   Any significant past or recent medical history: _____

_____

_____

_____

7   Name of diving supervisor: _____

8   Name of medical attendant: _____

9   Time of transmission of Part 1:   _____ GMT_____ Date

10   Addressee: _____

_____

11   Copied to: _____

_____

12   Telex confirmation sent at: _____ GMT_____ Date

13   Time message acknowledged: _____ GMT_____ Date

14   Reason for contacting shore doctor:

      Assistance required urgently

      Assistance required as soon as possible

      Assistance required when practicable

      Assistance required when patient gets ashore

      For information only

Part 2 Section B

Brief statement of the problem: _____

_____

_____

_____

_____

_____

_____

_____

_____

_____

Part 2 Section C

Summary of advice/instructions received from ashore: _____

_____

_____

_____

_____

_____

_____

_____

_____

Part 2 Section D

Details of treatment given (including therapeutic tables by number as well as depth, duration and

gases, and all supplementary therapy). State also times of implementation: _____

_____

_____

_____

_____

_____

_____

Part 2 Section E

Record of progress. Summary of history of the condition, with times of significant changes: _____

_____

_____

_____

_____

_____

_____

_____

_____

Part 2 Section F

Final outcome (e.g. fully recovered, transferred ashore under pressure etc.): _____

_____

_____

_____

_____

_____

_____

10

Part 3

RECORD OF MEDICAL EXAMINATION

All or part of this examination may be carried out at the request of the onshore doctor. Results should be recorded in the appropriate section and the questions which are not relevant to the particular incident left blank.

Part 3 Section A

EXAMINATION/GENERAL

1   Is the patient in pain? | YES | | NO |

     If 'yes', describe site, intensity and any factors which exacerbate or relieve it: _____

     _____

     _____

     _____

     _____

2   Has he any major injury? | YES | | NO |

     If 'yes', name the site and describe briefly. If there is bleeding give an estimate of blood loss:

     _____

     _____

     _____

     _____

     _____

3   What is his temperature?   _____ °C

4   Has he any skin rashes? | YES | | NO |

     If 'yes', describe appearance and site: _____

     _____

     _____

     _____

     _____

11

Part 3 Section B

CARDIORESPIRATORY SYSTEMS

5   Is his colour: Normal   [   ]

                      Pale   [   ]

                      Cyanosed (blue) [   ]

6   Is he sweating?   [YES]   [NO]

7   What is his: (i)   pulse_____ per minute

                     (ii)   blood pressure_____ Syst_____ Diast.

                     (iii)   respiratory rate_____ per minute

8   Does he have difficulty with breathing?   [YES]   [NO]

9   Does he have pain on breathing?   [YES]   [NO]

     If 'yes', describe: _____

     _____

     _____

     _____

10   Has he a cough?   [YES]   [NO]

         If 'yes', has he coughed blood?   [YES]   [NO]

11   Is he short of breath?   [YES]   [NO]

         If 'yes', has this been affected by:

         (i) increase of pressure   [YES]   [NO]

         (ii) decrease of pressure.   [YES]   [NO]

     If so, how? _____

     _____

     _____

12   Is the trachea (windpipe) central (i.e. normal)?   [YES]   [NO]

13   Is the apex (cardiac impulse) beat of the heart within 1" of the mid-
         clavicular line?   [YES]   [NO]

14   Are breath sounds audible equally on both sides of the chest?   [YES]   [NO]

12

15 Is there any subcutaneous emphysema (crackling sensation in tissues)?

YES NO

Part 3 Section C
ABDOMEN

16 Does the patient have abdominal pain?

YES NO

If 'yes', specify site by writing 16 on chart, and character: _____

_____

_____

_____

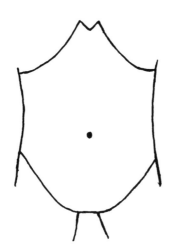

17 Does the patient have diarrhoea?

YES NO

18 Has the patient vomited?

YES NO

If 'yes': a) When did the patient last vomit? _____ GMT

b) If he is still vomiting, specify frequency and character: _____

_____

_____

13

19   Has he vomited blood? | YES | | NO |

20   Can the patient pass urine without difficulty? | YES | | NO |

21   Is the urine clear [   ] or blood stained [   ]

22   Is urinating painful? | YES | | NO |

23   Is the abdomen soft to palpation? | YES | | NO |

     If 'no', specify the site by writing 23 on chart

24   Are there any swellings in the abdomen? | YES | | NO |

     If 'yes', describe site (by writing 24 on chart), size and consistency _____

     _____

     _____

25   Can you hear bowel sounds? | YES | | NO |

Part 3 Section D
NERVOUS SYSTEM

26   Has he any visual disturbance? | YES | | NO |

     If 'yes', specify: _____

     _____

     _____

     _____

27   Has he a headache? | YES | | NO |

28   State of consciousness: Fully alert and orientated

                               Confused

                               Drowsy

                               Unconscious but responds to stimuli

                               Unconscious and unresponsive

29   Are pupils normal and equal in response to light? | YES | | NO |

If 'no', amplify: _____

_____

_____

30	Is the corneal (blink) reflex normal?	YES	NO
31	Does the patient have vertigo (dizziness)?	YES	NO
32	Does the patient have nystagmus (eye flickering)?	YES	NO
33	Is hearing equal and normal in both ears?	YES	NO

If 'no', specify: _____

_____

_____

_____

34   Are the remainder of the cranial nerves normal?

Eye movements	YES	NO	Swallowing reflex	YES	NO
Facial sensation	YES	NO	Tongue movement	YES	NO
Facial movement	YES	NO	Soft palate movement	YES	NO
Shrugging of shoulders	YES	NO			

35   Can the patient voluntarily move his:

R. Shoulder	YES	NO	L. Shoulder	YES	NO
R. Elbow	YES	NO	L. Elbow	YES	NO
R. Wrist	YES	NO	L. Wrist	YES	NO
R. Fingers	YES	NO	L. Fingers	YES	NO
R. Hip	YES	NO	L. Hip	YES	NO
R. Knee	YES	NO	L. Knee	YES	NO
R. Ankle	YES	NO	L. Ankle	YES	NO
R. Toes	YES	NO	L. Toes	YES	NO

36   Has he any weakness?   YES   NO

If 'yes', specify: _____

_____

_____

_____

37   Are reflexes (tendon jerks):   **Normal**   **Increased**   **Absent**   **?**

Triceps   R. ☐   ☐   ☐   ☐

L. ☐   ☐   ☐   ☐

Biceps   R. ☐   ☐   ☐   ☐

L. ☐   ☐   ☐   ☐

Knee   R. ☐   ☐   ☐   ☐

L. ☐   ☐   ☐   ☐

Ankle   R. ☐   ☐   ☐   ☐

L. ☐   ☐   ☐   ☐

38   Is the plantar response: ↑ R. ☐   ↑ L. ☐

OR   ↓ R. ☐   ↓ L. ☐

or not clear   R. ☐   L. ☐

39   Does he have 'pins and needles'?   ☐ YES   ☐ NO

If 'yes', specify: _____

_____

40   Is there a normal sensory response to pinprick?   ☐ YES   ☐ NO

If 'no', specify: _____

_____

Can you detect a level of sensory change?   ☐ YES   ☐ NO

41   Can he pass urine?   ☐ YES   ☐ NO

Part 3 Section E
ANY OTHER RELEVANT FINDINGS NOT LISTED ABOVE:

_____

_____

_____

_____

_____

Appendix 13

Sources of Assistance in Diving Emergencies

In the event of a diving emergency medical advice may be obtained from any of the following centres:

1. Offshore Medical Support, 12 Sunnybank Road, Aberdeen, AB2 3NG, Scotland

   For diving emergencies only: Aberdeen Aircall Number 871848
   Telex 73677 Casvac G Aberdeen

2. Aberdeen Industrial Doctors, 24 Albyn Place, Aberdeen, AB9 1RJ, Scotland

   Telephone: 24 hours Aberdeen (0224) 572879
   Telex 739148

3. North Sea Medical Centre, 3 Lowestoft Road, Gorleston-on-Sea, Great Yarmouth, Norfolk, NR31 6QB, England

   Telephone: During office hours Great Yarmouth (0493) 600011
   Other times Great Yarmouth (0493) 663264
   Telex: 975118 NOR MEDG

4. Duty Diving Officer, HMS Vernon, Portsmouth, Hants, England

   Telephone: Portsmouth (0705) 822351
   During working hours
   (Superintendent of Diving) Ext. HMS Vernon 22169 or 22782
   During non-working hours
   (Duty Lieutenant Commander) Ext. HMS Vernon 22008

5. London Medical Centre, 144 Harley Street, W1, England

   Telephone: During office hours 01-935-0023
   24 hours 01-274-3171

6. Fort Bovisand Emergency Service, Fort Bovisand, Plymouth, England

   Telephone: Plymouth (0752) 261910
   Ask for Duty Diving Doctor

7. Oil Duty Doctor Organisation (Offshore Emergency Medical Services), Norway

   Mobile telephone: 010 (Stavanger) 47-94-76700
   (As part of the Oil Duty Doctor Organisation's service, diving medical expertise is always provided)

8. Divers Alert Network (USA)
   Box 3823
   Duke University Medical Centre
   Durham, No. 27710

   Telephone: (919) 684 8111 (emergencies)
   (919) 684 2948 (information)

Appendix 14

Recommended Contents of First-Aid Boxes in Lifeboats and Survival Capsules

1. Tablets hyoscine 0.3 mg × 20
   Instructions — 2 tablets to be taken for seasickness. A further tablet can be taken every 4 hours
2. Parolein eye drops × 3 bottles
   Instructions — to be instilled in the eyes to remove oil or relieve salt water irritation
3. Tablets co-dydramol × 20
   Instructions — for relief of pain. Take 2 tablets every 4 hours
4. 1 set inflatable splints
5. 2 Guerdel airways
6. 2 Laerdal pocket masks
7. 4 Shell dressings
8. 6 cotton bandages 3 in.
9. 6 cotton bandages 2 in.
10. 6 triangular bandages
11. 6 packs of 4 in. square gauze (sterile; 5 per pack)
12. 3 eye pads
13. 1 pair scissors
14. 12 assorted safety pins
15. 1 packet cotton wool 250 g
16. Stretch fabric dressing strip 7.5 cm × 1 m
17. Elastic adhesive bandage BPC 7.5 cm × 4.5 m
18. TO BE PACKED IN A SEPARATE SEALED CONTAINER, WHICH SHOULD BE FIXED TO A BULKHEAD OR THE DECK:

    6 × 2 cc disposable sterile syringes with 6 × 23G 1¼-in. needles

    6 × 30 mg injections Pentazocine

    6 × 50 mg injections cyclizine

N.B. 6 × 15 mg injections morphine should also be kept in the installation's Controlled Drugs Cupboard, ready for putting in the lifeboat or survival capsule in the event of an 'abandon rig' situation.

Appendix 15

Recommended Furnishings and Equipment for Use in Hospitals on Offshore Installations

* These items will be required under the Offshore Installations and Pipeline Works (First-Aid) Regulations in United Kingdom Waters when they come into effect

Article	Special requirements	Quantities for installations or barges where the following numbers are regularly at work		
		1–25	26–100	101 or more
*Desk Writing platform	May be free-standing or wall mounted	1	1	1
*Telephone	A link into the barge/installation–shore line is essential. This phone link should also have capacity for use internally on the installation or barge	1	1	1
*Alarm bell system	The switch should be situated in the sick bay adjacent to the telephone. There should be repeater switches between each 2 beds. To obtain help quickly, it is suggested that an alarm should be in: (a) radio room; (b) control room (since these are usually occupied during all shifts); (c) medic's sleeping quarters so that he can be called at night (in this situation, the bell should be partly muted). A further switch should be fitted outside the sick bay to summon help quickly in the temporary absence of the medic			
*Filing cabinet	Four-drawer with locks for retention of record cards		1	1
*Cabinet	Lockable and refrigerated, for retention of medications	1	1	1
*Accident record book		1	1	1
*Daily treatment record book		1	1	1
*Language interpretation cards	In appropriate languages for those on the installation or barge	1	1	1
*Mirror			1	1

Article	Special requirements	Quantities for installations or barges where the following numbers are regularly at work		
		1–25	26–100	101 or more
*Angle-poise lamp	Wall mounted			
	Free-standing	1	1	1
*Chairs	Tubular steel and padded	1	2	2
*Examination chair	With adjustable head rest and pedal-operated moveable back rest		1	1
*Armchair	Padded, washable covering		1	1
*Footstool	Adjustable, steel. Painted and/or chrome finish		1	1
*Dressing bin	Chrome or stainless finish. Pedal-operated, disposable inner lining	1	1	1
*Bed and mattress	Mobile hospital type bed with brakes and tilt facilities, 6 × 3 ft. Mattress to be covered in waterproof material		2	2
*Sheets	See following entry		10	20
*Blankets	Cellular cotton. Duvets may be used as alternatives and if so should be fitted with washable covers. If these are used quantities of sheets may be adjusted			
	Blankets	6	18	24
	Duvets		6	12
	Duvet covers		9	16
*Pillows	Filled with non-flammable foam and with washable covers and waterproof inner covering			
	Pillows	2	6	12
	Covers	3	9	16
*Plastic sheets	Disposable, suggested size 2 × 5 ft.		100	200
*Screen curtains	Each 3 × 6 ft., washable and fitted with securing hoods		12	20
Examination couch	Or minor operating table	1	1	1
Storage cabinet	For drugs and dressings	1	1	1
Portable operating light	For use off mains or battery		1	1
*Screen curtain ceiling track	Fitted so that each bed is individually screened		As required	
*Bedside locker	May be free-standing or hinged to wall		2	2
*Bed light	To be fitted over each bed on ceiling or wall (bright/dim switch to be operated at bedside)		2	2
Dressing trolley	Stainless steel	1	1	1
Aspirator	Electric		1	1
Emergency lights	Battery-operated, hand-held, high-luminosity lights	1	2	3
Scales	To weigh to 100 kg	1	1	1
Drip stand		1	1	1
Lockable cabinet	Double-locked cabinet for storage of controlled drugs	1	1	1

Subject Index

Note: The term 'offshore' is used in this index for clarification purposes only. All entries, unless otherwise qualified, refer to offshore situations, etc.